With my warm

Kitty Little:

Kitty Little's Book of Herbal Beauty

Kitty Little's

Book of Herbal Beauty

Illustrated by John Dodson

Jill Norman

Jill Norman Ltd
90 Great Russell Street, London WC1B 3PY
Published in association with Penguin Books Ltd

First published 1980

Printed and bound in Great Britain
by W & J Mackay Ltd, Chatham
Designed by Ken Garland and Associates

British Library Cataloguing in Publication Data

Little, Kitty
Kitty Little's book of herbal beauty.
1. Beauty, Personal 2. Herbs
I. Book of herbal beauty
646. 7′2 RA778
ISBN 0–906908–01–9

To Martin, who gives me the freedom of his heart

Some of them will saye, seeing that I graunte that I have gathered this booke of so manye writers, that I offer unto you an heape of other mennis laboures, and nothinge of myne owne . . . To whom I annsere that if the honye that the bees gather out of so manye floure of herbes, shrubbes, and trees, that are growing in other mennis meadowes, feldes and closes may justelye be called the bee's honye . . . So maye I call it that I have learned and gathered of manye good autoures . . . my booke.

William Turner

Contents

List of illustrations

Black and White Illustrations

Colour Plates (between pp 112 and 113)

Acknowledgements

I am indebted to Jill Norman, my editor, who has mastered the gentle art of constructive criticism so well she almost made me feel I had arrived at her intelligent viewpoint all by myself. My thanks to Jim Paton who willingly embarked on the first reading of this book.

Thanks, too, to Anne Soan, my secretary, who typed a meticulous copy of the final draft and who managed to retain her infectious sense of enthusiasm throughout, and to Muriel Watterson who helped me construct the index.

Marjorie Leese, whose gardening experience has proved invaluable, helped me grow all the herbs mentioned in this book and many more. Mr and Mrs Hugo, who own the Ashfield Herb Nursery, gladly contributed some of the herbs used for the illustrations as well as many of those I grow for my own experiments. John Dodson has produced illustrations which are so beautifully accurate they exceeded even my exacting expectations. Frank Dellicompagni, my hairdresser, read through the section on hair and Mr P R Walker and Mr A P Bell looked at the section on dental care. Thank you all.

I am grateful to Keele University where I studied for my PhD, who welcomed me back and gave me a corner of peace in which to write; to the British Library and to Kew Gardens where I spent many happy hours enjoying the contents of the gardens as well as their library facilities.

Lastly, I am truly grateful to Ann and Dennis Smith who lent me their cottage in Yorkshire which provided me with an oasis of calm in which to complete the book. I hope both the peace and the enthusiasm so many friends contributed shines through the following pages.

Introduction

I was not born with a herbal sprig in my mouth instead of the proverbial silver spoon. Nor has my family hoarded beauty secrets that have been passed down to me from generations back. My interest in herbs and in the way in which they can be used to achieve a harmonious balance between serenity, vitality and beauty crept up on me over a period of several years. It began with seemingly endless afternoons spent in the British Museum researching for my doctoral thesis in quite a different subject. When I tired of this I used to revive my flagging spirits by browsing through old herbals and manuscripts, some of them dating back to Anglo-Saxon times. They contained a cornucopia of herbal recipes liberally laced with extravagant superstitions, herbal folklore, religious philosophy and plenty of sage and witty advice about survival tactics for life in general. I found the mixture irresistible.

I began to experiment with some of the more likely sounding concoctions said to care for the body using the herbs in my garden that I had hitherto only considered for culinary use. Whatever else their faults the old herbalists were certainly not interested in dull exactitude so the results were sometimes disastrous and often hilarious. But a few of them were startlingly successful. I discovered that certain herbs, used by themselves or combined with other natural foods, performed all the functions of commercially made cosmetics, but they did so more gently, more naturally and, I was finally convinced, far more effectively than their synthetic, chemical-laden modern counterparts. Herbs were able to moisturize, cleanse, disinfect, soothe, heal, lubricate, stimulate and refine the skin. I found they could also be used internally to encourage a healthy skin, strong nails and shining eyes and hair. No herb worked miracles overnight but the results were good enough to encourage me to grow a more adventurous selection of them. I was then lucky enough to rent a house from a delightful lady who not only shared my fascination with herbs but who also owned four acres of land on which to grow them. The herb garden we encouraged has become a perpetual pleasure, a sanctuary of fragrance, sunlight and tranquillity where even the humblest of the wild herbs that are often mistakenly spurned as weeds have their own special place.

After several years of trial and not a little error my experiments with herbs blossomed into a business which produces skin care products and pot pourris following as closely as possible the recipes I gleaned in the British Museum. Of course, there have had to be changes. We are no longer living in the age of the Elizabethan still-room in which the mistress of the house concocted ointments, medicines, sweet waters and washing balls for her household's use from the herbs she had culled in her garden. My company now exports our products to many parts of the world and I have not been averse to using modern cosmetic techniques, providing they improve the quality or the efficacy of the product.

This book is the result of that compromise: a blending of the original spirit of the old herbals, stripped of their vagaries and superstition, together with modern knowledge about dermatology, trichology, dentistry and cosmetic manufacturing techniques. The first chapter will tell you how to process herbs for cosmetic use, the last one how to grow them. The space in between is filled with recipes which are as sound and as pertinent today as they were three or thirteen hundred years ago, recipes which I hope will encourage beauty which is more than skin-deep. Happiness starts in the soul and floods outwards. Internal contentment works wonders for the exterior, which is why I have included a chapter on how to cope with emotional stress and distress using natural remedies.

I am not a doctor, a cosmetician, a scientist or even a qualified herbalist. I have been described as a renaissance lady, meaning I have an unbounded curiosity about everything, coupled with an enthusiastic ability to turn my discoveries to practical use. That is all this book requires of you. You will find following the recipes as easy as using a cookery book. Do not be deterred by the fact that many of the herbs mentioned sound esoteric. It is possible to grow them all yourself and many of them can be bought. Appendix II, (p. 232) contains useful names and addresses which will help you find suppliers of everything you will need.

Most herbs are enormously versatile and you will find that nearly all parts of a herb can be put to good use and have several functions. Take great mullein, for example. It is a tall,

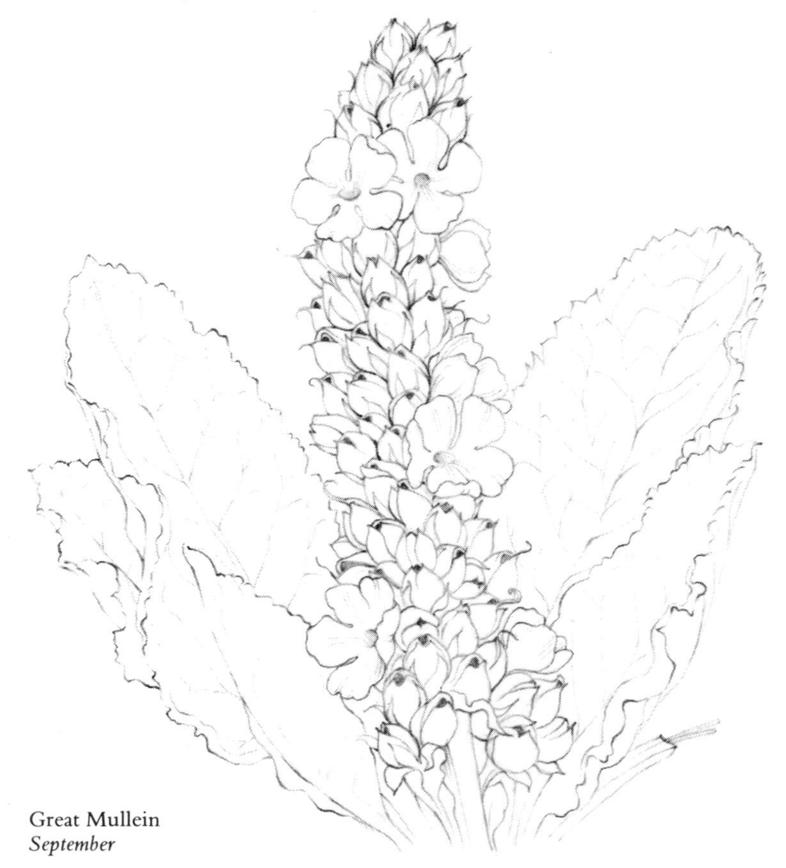

Great Mullein
September

stately-looking herb whose yellow flowers have been used for hundreds of years to tint hair Titian gold, to cure earache, piles, sprains, gout and bed wetting. Its thick soft leaves have been used to line the soles of thin shoes; wrapped round sore throats and mouths throbbing with toothache; dried and smoked to relieve pulmonary congestion, and also as a gentle sedative. Its root has been used to remove warts and relieve migraine and its seeds have been used by poachers to intoxicate fish and as a poultice to draw out splinters. In view of their versatility I have prepared a long list of herbs specially selected for each particular skin and hair type, leaving the choice to you, according to their availability and your own preferences.

Sadly, our lives now seem to be dominated by convenient pre-packaged products and persuasive advertising. We have replaced the peace and the leisure of recipes which instruct you to stir while you measure time by saying 'the Misere Psalm very slowly' or 'about an Ave Maria while' with strident bells and automatic oven timers. We have deadened our senses to the real look, feel, smell and taste of herbs and natural foods by filling ourselves with synthetic additives and preservatives, and by bombarding our skins with chemicals and various ingredients that have been extracted from or used on animals cruelly. Yet, as this book will show you, herbs and various other natural foods offer pleasant and effective alternatives. Some of the good herbs will do you lies in the simple pleasurable act of their gathering. Immersing yourself in the sunlit beauty and fragrance of a herb garden is only the beginning of the complete pleasure of making your own natural cosmetics. Once appropriated, the delights of herbalism will last in you like the scent of woodruff which grows stronger as it grows older.

Chapter 1
Using Herbs

The Anglo-Saxon word for herb was *wèod*, which we have corrupted to 'weed', and it is as well to remember that many of the plants we tear out of our gardens and throw away today were originally used as herbs. They were either long-established wildings or survivors from earlier deliberate introductions which got out of hand and rampaged over the surrounding area. Ground elder, for example, was first introduced into Britain in the Middle Ages as a cure for gout but it spread so quickly that it was nicknamed 'Jack-jump-about', and it has now worn out its welcome in most gardens. So think of nettles, cleavers, chickweed, clover, coltsfoot, daisies, dandelions, ground elder, ivy, horsetail, thistles and yarrow not as weeds but as wild herbs. As with cultivated herbs, make sure before gathering that they are not contaminated by carbon monoxide fumes, or the various chemical sprays and powders farmers use to fertilize their crops and kill weeds. I never pick any wild herbs growing near roadsides and in railway cuttings, nor will I use those that grow on the edges of large cultivated fields. I avoid picking herbs which are yellowed, faded, wilted, mottled or insect-eaten.

Fresh herbs are preferable and superior to dried ones, which inevitably lose some of their characteristic smell and taste no matter how meticulous the drying process has been. Basil is one that springs immediately to mind. Its pungent peppery scent when fresh is subdued to a mere dusty hint of its former glory when dried. The only herbs of which this is not true are woodruff and elderflowers. Fresh woodruff is almost odourless; it only starts emitting its delightful new-mown hay fragrance once it is dried and the older it gets the more the fragrance increases – up to a point, of course. Elderflowers tend to smell quite rancid until they are processed to produce elderflower water and essential oil.

The essential oils, which are the odoriferous substances in herbs, are delicate and ethereal and some do tend to get lost in the drying. This is unfortunate because not only do they increase the production of white corpuscles if taken internally but, used externally, they improve the circulation of blood to the skin and some of them encourage perspiration, help soothe inflammation and are highly effective bactericides and disinfectants. Lavender oil is one of the best known antiseptics and was used extensively during the last war to fight infection in wounds. It was also used to purify surgical dressings.

All the recipes in this book require fresh herbs unless dried herbs are specifically mentioned. But do not despair if you have not got the room, the energy or the inclination to cultivate your own cosmetic herbs: you can still gather wild herbs or buy small quantities of cultivated ones. Dried herbs, as long as they are carefully *green dried* (meaning as long as they do not look sad, dusty and grey, yellow or bleached) are acceptable substitutes. They are also, of course, far more convenient in the winter when only the hardy woody herbs continue to flourish. Dried herbs are more concentrated and so quantities will have to be reduced accordingly. The guide on p. 24 will help you in this respect.

How to Identify your Herbs

The illustrations will help you to identify the herbs you will need, but obviously it has not been possible to show them all, so I have included a list of all the herbs mentioned in this book together with their botanical names (see p. 228). A book primarily intended for plant identification will be invaluable – the ones I have found particularly helpful are listed in the bibliography. The herbs illustrated in this book were all taken from my own herb garden or from my local herb farm between August and December. Bear this in mind when you are trying to identify them at other times of the year and if in doubt about the identity of a herb do not pick it. Hemlock, for example, looks remarkably like parsley to the untutored and its root has been mistaken for parsnip, its seeds for anise.

Protected Species

In 1975 parliament passed The Conservation of Wild Creatures and Wild Plants Act, which states that it is a criminal offence to dig up any British wild plant, no matter how common it might be, without the consent of the owner of the land on which it grows. The twenty most rare plants in Britain cannot even be picked, according to the Act, and a list of them can be obtained from the Conservation Department, Royal Botanic Gardens, Kew, Surrey. Do try and remember that some plants, and this includes herbs, only grow in certain areas, so if you dig them up you may be destroying their habitat forever.

Gathering Herbs

Do not choose herbs which grow tightly packed in clumps and which are fighting for soil and air space. Well-spaced herbs will be better nourished and consequently better for you. Never strip an area of any one herb. Be selective. A few herbs judiciously picked at intervals will ensure the same herb is available next year for even annuals, if allowed to come to seed, can replant themselves.

Herb gathering is a meticulous art. Herbs should be picked at exactly the right moment when their various qualities are at their peak, at what the seventeenth-century herbalists used to call the 'balsamic moment'. For most herbs, this is usually during the late spring and summer, in the early morning, once the dew has evaporated, or in the late afternoon. Dew-wet or rain-wet herbs are prone to mildew. Flowers that you intend to pick should be left unwatered the day before you pick them.

Leaves should be picked young, just before the flowers open, when the leaf shoots contain concentrated medicinal powers.

Nipping them will also help the plant to thicken up.

Flowers are fragile and should be gathered the moment they open, before they have been pollinated. This way their essential oils will remain in the petals instead of being exuded into the air. Try not to handle the petals at all. Hold the blooms by the stalks and snip these off directly over a drying tray or a flat basket so that the petals can fall on to it untouched.

Seeds should be allowed to enjoy the sun as long as possible but keep an eye on them to make sure they are not blown away by the wind. Cut the seed-laden branches and hang them upside down over a tray or a box which will catch the seeds as they fall. Keep different bunches of herbs well apart so that the falling seeds do not become muddled. Sometimes, during especially dry summers, it is possible to let the seeds dry on the plant itself, but this has its disadvantages because the longer the seeds stay out the more chance there is of the wind dispersing them while you are not looking.

Most seeds can be kept for years before planting but, as with all generalizations, there are always exceptions. Angelica seed loses its germinating power very quickly so seeds should really be planted within several days of their ripening on the parent plant. If you do have some old angelica seeds don't throw them away. Sprinkle them on to a low fire and they will fill the house with a delightful fragrance.

Barks and roots should be gathered in the spring and autumn when they are thick and juicy with sap.

Lift roots out carefully without cutting or bruising them, shake them free of soil, cut off any little hair rootlets and wash well under running water. Dry carefully with a tea towel. Only strip bark off the larger branches of well-established trees. If you try this with saplings you may kill them.

Berries should be picked well before they have any chance to turn mushy. The use of a fork makes the stripping of small juicy berries, such as elderberries, easier.

Equipment for Collecting Herbs

Never collect herbs in plastic bags, which will only heat them up and trap any traces of moisture on them, so speeding up their deterioration. Choose instead a big, flat, woven rose basket which will allow you to separate and keep track of your herbs and prevent them from becoming crushed, bruised and otherwise damaged.

Handle herbs gently and as briefly as possible. Pluck the leaves off with your fingers and, if you have to use a knife, scissors or even secateurs for the woodier, tougher herbs be as quick and as precise as you can. Some metals, especially aluminium, tend to taint herbs with their taste or to stain them.

Drying

Take your freshly picked herbs indoors as quickly as possible. Sort them, lay them out or hang them in small bunches. Herbs should always be dried in the warmest, driest, airiest, darkest conditions you can create. This is particularly important; poorly dried herbs are as bad as no herbs at all. Strong sunlight and wind will only leach the herb of its valuable essential oils.

An airing cupboard is ideal for drying in small quantities. Make screens by covering wooden frames with nylon netting or, better still, cheesecloth, as I believe herbs prefer to come into contact only with natural substances. My feeling about this is purely intuitive; I can offer no visible proof except to say that herbs I have dried on wire netting or even on nylon appear duller in colour and seem to have less fragrance than those dried on cotton. Tack the fabric tightly round the sides. Old picture frames are ideal for this purpose because they are generally fairly thick (anything thicker than 2 cm (¾ in.) wide will do), will not buckle and can be stacked on top of each other, leaving space for the warm air to circulate freely between the layers. During the course of the first few days turn the herbs over frequently so that they dry evenly.

Woodier herbs can be tied in *small* bunches and hung from hooks in a warm dry room. I emphasize that the bunches should be kept small because large bunches will block the free circulation of air through them so the herbs start warming up in the middle of the bunch and rotting from the inside out. I hang my lavender, woodruff, rosemary, sage, tansy and thyme from the beams in my kitchen. Of course, herbs should never be hung in a spot where steam and condensation from cooking or laundering will get to them. Nor should they be dried in garages, however warm. Having taken some trouble to gather chemical-free herbs you will hardly want them choked with exhaust fumes.

Some authorities recommend oven drying but I have always found this method far too harsh for most herbs. Fragile leaves and flowers and even seeds tend to emerge singed and brown simply because it it so difficult to control the temperature of the oven, which should never exceed 32°C (90°F). Leaving the oven door partly open will help keep the temperature down. Oven drying is fairly satisfactory for hardy roots and barks and may even be imperative in cold climates where, if the drying is too prolonged, the plant starts to rot.

Drying roots and barks can be speeded up by cutting roots in slivers and peeling bark into thin strips. This has the added advantage of making them easier to use as it is very difficult to cut up or even pound well-dried roots and barks. Once they break and crack sharply when they are bent you can be sure they are quite dry. If they are still pliable and will only bend, or if they are leathery and still have spongy or fibrous cores, they need further drying time.

Seeds should be stirred from time to time and once they crack between your fingernails, they are thoroughly dried. Leaves and stalks are dry when they feel crisp and crackly to the touch; petals are dry when they lose their silky texture and feel paper thin.

Storing Dried Herbs

Separate the leaves from any remaining stalks and, if you want them powdered, rub them between your hands. Powdered herbs have few advantages for cosmetic use, except in face masks, poultices and alcoholic macerations. They will not dissolve in liquid and whole herbs at least can be easily strained out of liquids, so I keep few powdered herbs. Finely powdered herbs also tend to go stale more quickly than whole ones and it makes my hands very sore rubbing any quantity of herbs between them. (If you must powder them they respond better to this kindly treatment than to being forced through the mesh of a sieve.) You can pound the whole herb with a pestle and mortar but this method is not recommended for the woodier herbs as their stalks are very hard to pulverize. Preparing powdered herbs also tends to clog up the lungs and the throat so wear a smog mask to protect yourself from their fine dust. This is a simple but very effective gauze covering for the nose and mouth which can be bought at a chemist's shop. Do not throw away the twigs of the more aromatic herbs. Instead, tie them in bundles and add them to open log fires or to a barbecue grill. Lavender stalks can be burnt like joss sticks to perfume the air. Why not try reviving the dainty medieval English custom of serving small dessert fruits or sweets speared by lavender sticks?

The fruits of your labours should ideally be stored away from direct light in green or amber glass jars with ground glass stoppers or corks which will seal in their fragrance (one of the surest tests of a well-dried herb apart from its greenness is how fresh it smells). Nothing damages dried herbs more than exposure to heat, sunlight or damp. If they are stored in damp conditions it only needs a tiny part to get mildewed before the mildew spreads and ruins all your efforts. Light and heat simply extract the active principles of the herbs and fritter them away into the surrounding air, and you have more need of them. Label and date each jar clearly as soon as the herb is inside. This will prevent any muddle later on when you come to use them. Renew your stocks of dried herbs yearly and treat your compost heap to the residue. The only exceptions to this rule are barks and roots which can be stored for two years before use. If you have to use clear glass containers, wrap a nice big label around them to protect them from the light. Store all your herbs in a dark, dry cupboard or, failing this, the darkest corner of your kitchen or pantry. So much for those pretty kitchen herb racks with their clear glass jars and exposed shelves!

Never store herbs in plastic bags, which noticeably alter the constituents of the herb, and try to avoid paper bags if possible – they are not sufficient protection against mildew, insects and mice. Anyway, darkened glass jars enable you to check the level of your herb and how well it is keeping at a glance. If you do see a few beads of moisture in the jar within the first few days do not panic. This simply means that in spite of all your precautions the herb is not sufficiently dried. Just empty out the herbs on to the drying tray, dry again and make sure your glass container is dry too when you bottle up the herbs a second time.

Try to use any fresh herbs as quickly as possible but if you have to store them keep them in a jar with an airtight lid in the fridge. There are two other ways of preserving herbs, which have their limited cosmetic uses.

Salting Herbs

Some herbs, like basil, marjoram, thyme, rosemary, lavender, sage, tansy and the mints, take quite well to this traditional Indian method of preservation. Pack a wide-necked preserving jar with alternate layers of leaves on their stalks and coarse sea salt, finishing with a thick covering of salt. Cover closely with a round of greaseproof paper and seal tightly. When you want to use the herb simply shake the sprig free of salt and wash under running water.

Herbs with Salt and Oil

Follow the same process as above but sprinkle each layer of herb with equal quantities of coarse sea salt and vegetable oil. The whole mixture can be used strained or unstrained as a herbal body rub. The unstrained oil is messy but fun. It is advisable to rub some into your forearm first to test it. Some of the darker herbs may leave a slight green stain on your skin and you do not want to look like the proverbial Martian. Strained oils will not stain your skin.

Freezing Herbs

This method is really only recommended as a stop-gap as it destroys some of the properties necessary for cosmetic and medicinal use. However, I have found it quite a convenient way of making herbal pouchettes for the bath with something resembling fresh herbs in the middle of winter. First make sure the herbs are clean and moisture-free. Snip them up into small wax containers, close them, label and freeze. When you want to use them simply take the carton out of the freezer and leave the contents to defrost in it. They will certainly have lost something of their former glory but they will still be quite usable.

Never wrap herbs in foil or in plastic bags before freezing. Aluminium may discolour them and in my experience plastic seems to destroy the vitality of the herb.

Equipment for Herbal Preparation

You will need kitchen scales which will measure small quantities accurately but, as many fresh herbs are bulky, scales with a large weighing pan are helpful. The mini-balances sold by some home-brewing shops may also be useful. Where the amount of herbs required is so small that it is impossible to measure it accurately I have given the measurement in teaspoons or tablespoons. For your guidance, 5 g ($^1/_6$ oz) is approximately equivalent to one level tablespoon of dried herbs. A few glass, china or pottery bowls, a palette knife with a flexible blade, a measuring jug, an eyedropper, plenty of self-adhesive labels and a pestle and mortar are also essential. Teaspoons, tablespoons, measuring jugs, scales, knives and sieves should be anything but aluminium. Start collecting glass, not plastic, jars and bottles of all shapes and sizes, together with their caps or stoppers. Very small glass bottles with necks that are not too narrow are particularly useful for storing your essential herbal oils. You will need an eyedropper for measuring out tiny quantities of these essential oils. The palette knife is useful for scraping out every bit of herb and the bowls for mixing or to use as the top part of a double boiler for melting honey, lanolin or waxes. A porcelain saucepan in which to make your emulsions is the ultimate luxury and can be used instead of a double boiler. Emulsions can be beaten with a sterilized birch twig whisk which does not scratch the saucepan, but remember anything porcelain must be protected by a heat diffusing mat so that it does not crack. This type of saucepan retains heat particularly well so use only the most moderate amount of heat and draw the saucepan off the stove as soon as the waxes and oils have melted. Try and invest in a pestle and mortar which is solid and heavy: herbs need weight behind them to be crushed and the flimsy wooden pestles and mortars which seem to be increasingly in vogue merely bounce over the table as you pound. Glass ones may look beautiful but they scratch very easily and I keep worrying about where all that finely gouged-out glass goes to, except into my herbs. My own mortar is a Japanese one called a *suribachi*. It is made of stoneware with thin grooves running in wedge shapes set at various angles inside a bowl. These grooves give the mortar a special edge over the conventional ones, making it magnificently efficient. The mortar is then easily cleaned with a birch twig brush. Suribachis can be bought in Japanese gift shops and you may find them in wholefood stores.

An electric beater and a blender are useful but not essential as is an electric or hand-turned coffee grinder. Two sieves are needed, one large and one small, through which to strain your herbal tea. Some sort of filtering system is essential, such as big squares of muslin or cheesecloth or, better still, coffee filter papers. They may be too small for filtering major efforts such as large brews for a herbal bath but they are satisfactory for most other tasks. They strain out even the finest powdered herb, can be squeezed out to extract the last drop of goodness from an infusion and then thrown away. Cheesecloth and muslin have to be washed constantly and getting every last trace of herb out can sometimes prove difficult. They also need to be sterilized by boiling, which is tedious.

How Much to Use

You do not have to be too rigid about the quantities of herb you use, but this reassurance does not give you licence to go mad. The old adage 'a little of what you fancy does you good' is particularly true of herbs but you could poison yourself by using large quantities, at least internally. You would have some difficulty poisoning yourself with their external use unless you actually applied a poisonous herb.

One real difficulty will probably be with the sheer bulk of fresh herbs which will not sit on a kitchen scale obediently, so for your guidance all the woodier herbs dry out to about a quarter of their original weight; the fleshy ones containing larger quantities of water dry out to about a twentieth of their fresh weight; petals, roots and barks all dry out to about a tenth of their fresh weight. One big cupped handful of dried herbs generally weighs about 30 g (1 oz) and is equivalent to three big cupped handfuls of the same fresh material.

Herbs in Food and Drink

The old herbals, if they mention quantities at all, do so very rarely and in the same spirit with which I tend to cook – a pinch of this and a handful of that. If any herbs are dangerous I have said so and stated exact quantities and the frequency of use. Pay special attention to these instructions and treat all herbs with respect. Taken as medicines or used externally they will certainly not wreak the same havoc as their chemical counterparts. Instead, they will work slowly but surely and so gently that many people used to the stronger onslaughts of chemicals may not even notice their effect at first. Persistence is the key to their cosmetic use. Do not expect to follow a herbal skin care routine tonight and look like Candice Bergen or Alain Delon (depending on your sex and your aspirations) tomorrow. The same is true of herbs for culinary use. Herbs used in food and drinks are just as important as herbs used externally. After all, you function as a whole and external beauty is utterly dependent on the proper working of all bodily functions. Start looking after your skin from the inside out by including herbs in your diet. Nearly all the herbs you apply externally will do you just as much good if you ingest them.

Probably the most effective way of getting all the goodness out of any herb is to eat or drink it. The Elizabethans used to decorate their salads with rose petals, borage flowers, primroses, cowslips, carnations, violets, rosemary, sage, angelica, nasturtiums, viper's bugloss, lavender, marigolds, elderflowers and orange blossom. They boiled roots of angelica, rampion, parsnip, daisy, elecampane or they pickled them and added them cold and sliced. They used leaves and buds from the most unlikely plants: ash keys, broom buds, plantain, yarrow, mallow, purslane, hyssop, rocket, ox-eye daisy leaves, tansy and even vine tendrils. How unimaginative our salads now seem compared to those artistic triumphs. They made drinks, hypocras, wines, caudles, metheglin and non-alcoholic cordial waters from almost every herb available whether it was wild or cultivated, and salep, the root of the orchis, was still in vogue in the eighteenth century as a drink. At one time it even rivalled the popularity of coffee and there was a salep house in Fleet Street. It was reputed to be an aphrodisiac but fell from grace either because it did not work or because the taste and texture made it unpalatable (it had to be mixed with wine to make it drinkable). So be imaginative and experiment with the herbs you use in food and in drinks.

Roasted dandelion roots can be ground and used to make a milder version of ordinary coffee. Some herb seeds are rather nice to crunch just by themselves. Dill and fennel used to be eaten during boring Sunday sermons to while away the time and suppress mounting hunger pangs. Those herbs that are generally unpalatable eaten raw can be taken in an infusion and sweetened with honey. Admittedly, a taste for herbal tea is something that has to be acquired (rather like learning to enjoy the subtleties of a good wine) but once acquired there will be no holding you. You will find yourself foisting spicy hibiscus punch and juniper berry tea on to disbelieving friends and revelling in the rare distinction of being a herbal tea connoisseur instead of a wine buff.

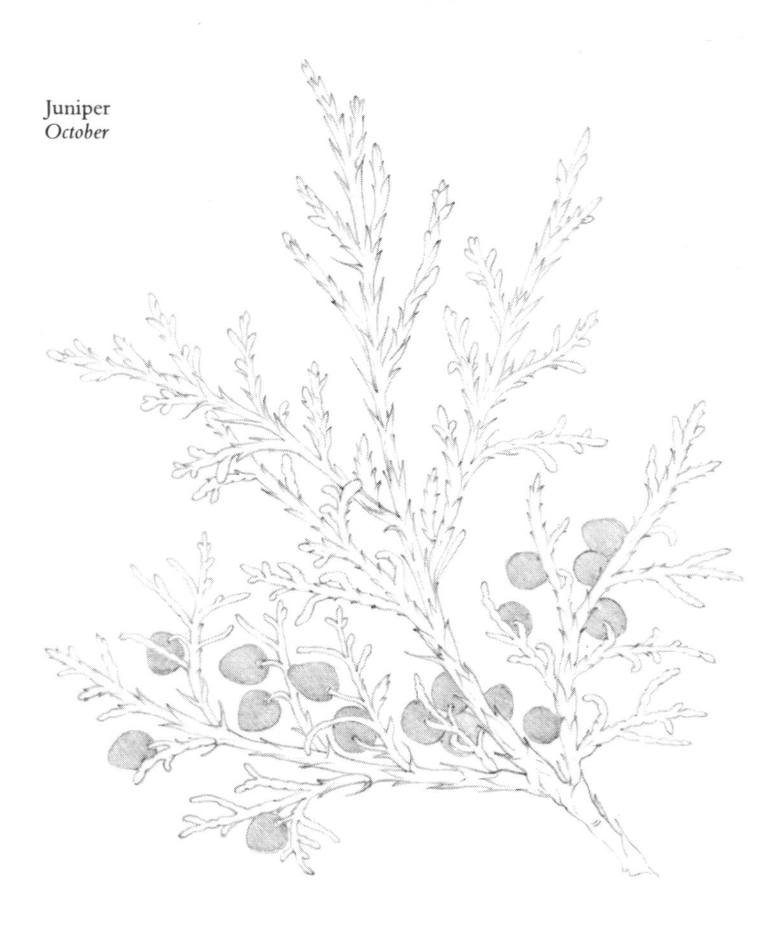
Juniper
October

Herbal Tea

Any metal will contaminate and destroy a herb's delicate flavour so use only china, pottery, porcelain, unchipped enamel or glass as vessels in which to make an infusion. Keep a teapot aside specially for herbal teas if you can. Ordinary teapots tend to get stained with tannin and this ruins the delicate flavour of herbal teas as does steeping the herbs too long. If you are using particularly delicate herbs such as sweet cicely or elderflowers, rather than risk steeping them too long increase the quantity of the herb. Make herbal tea exactly as you would ordinary tea, using one teaspoon of dried herbs for every person and one for the pot. Alternatively, use three times the amount of fresh herb, first bruising the leaves slightly with a pestle and mortar. Begin by warming the pot, add the requisite quantity of herbs, pour boiling water over them, cover tightly and leave to brew for five to ten minutes. Strain, remembering to use a nylon not a metal sieve. If you prefer iced teas, let the brew cool and then strain and refrigerate. Iced teas should be allowed to brew five minutes longer than usual as their flavour needs to be accentuated when cold.

To make a seed tea bruise the seeds with a pestle and mortar, pour boiling water into an enamel saucepan, add the bruised seed and bring to the boil. Simmer gently for five to ten minutes. Strain and serve immediately. Be adventurous about your herbal teas. Try marrying the flavours. Hibiscus and rosehip are a perfect match, and a rose geranium leaf slightly crushed and added to lemon balm tea heightens both its fragrance and its flavour. The duller teas like horsetail and yarrow can be mixed with the more positive flavour of any of the mints.

Infusion

An infusion is made in exactly the same way as a tea only it is somewhat stronger. Use 30 g (1 oz) of the dried herb or a handful and a quarter of fresh herb to a litre (1 ¾ pints) of water. It can be stored in a glass container covered with a piece of linen or muslin in the refrigerator for three days. After this it may start fermenting and should be thrown away. You can tell when it does – fine bubbles start to pop up to the surface.

Decoction

This again is made in the same way as a herbal tea but is usually made from seeds, roots or barks, which tend, because of their toughness, to need more rigorous processing in order to induce them to give up their properties. Use 30 g (1 oz) of dried or fresh seeds, dried root or bark. Fresh roots should be used in the case of valerian (for detailed instructions on how to make valerian tea, see p. 205). Simmer the herb in a partly covered enamel saucepan for twenty minutes or until your litre (1¾ pints) of water is reduced to approximately half the quantity. Decoctions can occasionally be made from leaves if a stronger result is required but this method should not be used on flowers. To make a double-strength infusion or decoction simply double the amount of herb used and keep to the same quantity of water as for a single-strength mixture. To make a quadruple-strength infusion or decoction increase the original amount of herb used four times and use the same quantity of water as for a single-strength mixture.

Herb Milk

Milk is very good at absorbing the essential oils from herbs. Simply chop up a cupped handful of fresh herbs and stir them into half a litre (1 pint) of milk. Cover with muslin or a piece of linen and leave the mixture to stand for at least four hours. Strain through a nylon sieve, mashing the herb hard with a wooden spoon to wring out the last of its juices. The milk will have taken on the colour of the herb you are using. Fresh flower petals can be treated in the same way, using a handful to half a litre (1 pint) of milk. This method works best with fresh herbs but dried herbs can be effectively macerated in milk which has first been well heated but not allowed to boil. Stir 30 g (1 oz) of dried herb into half a litre (1 pint) of warm milk and proceed as above. This method is not recommended for seeds, barks, dried flower petals and most types of root, though orchis root is still drunk in the Middle East, mixed with half-and-half quantities of warm milk and water and flavoured with spices.

Maceration

Water, oil, cider vinegar or white wine vinegar, wine, vodka, brandy and gin are all suitable liquids in which to macerate herbs. The results, depending on which you use, are all given different names.

Water maceration is not often used as, not surprisingly, it tends to be a rich breeding ground for bacteria. It can be quite successful as a way to make garden fertilizer (see Chapter 8) or to extract the fragrance from flowers. Indeed it was this method, so legend has it, that first resulted in rose oil when the marriage of an Indian princess to an emperor in 1612 was celebrated in luxurious and extravagant style. The canal on which the royal barge floated was filled with rose petals and when the princess languidly dangled her hand in the water she noticed an oily layer had collected on it. This oil was carefully skimmed off and used and is said to have been the original attar of roses. You can create the same effect (somewhat more prosaically) by strewing an enamel or earthenware casserole dish with 3 cm (1¼ in.) of the reddest, most fragrant rose petals you can find and covering them with 4 cm (1½ in.) of water. Put the dish out into the sun and cover with a piece of cling film to prevent insects jumping in. In this instance muslin will not do as it blocks the sun's rays. Leave it undisturbed for three days. You will then notice an oily iridescence floating on the surface. Collect this with cotton wool swabs which should be squeezed out into a wide-necked amber or green glass bottle. Leave the bottle in turn out in the sun, this time completely open, until the water evaporates. Do not expect the result to be as strong as real attar of roses: it takes nearly thirty whole roses to make just one drop of the real thing. Decant your precious few teaspoons of oil into a tiny bottle and cover tightly.

Essential oil is easy to make and the result is most satisfying. Pound up one cupped handful of the fresh herb with a pestle and mortar until it is a green mulch. Scrape this into a large preserving jar and cover with half a litre (1 pint) of any vegetable oil of your choice. (I always use sweet almond oil in my company's products as it yields the finest results but corn oil and groundnut oil are cheaper.) Add a tablespoon of cider vinegar. Close tightly or, if you are using a preserving jar, vacuum seal with the lid. Make sure the jar is only about three quarters full so there is room to shake the mixture vigorously.

Do this and then put outside in the strong sunlight. Shake the jar hard whenever you pass it or think about it. In about a month the oil should be ready for straining through a nylon sieve. Mash the herbs well into the sieve during this process to extract every last drop of the oil but if it is not strong enough simply repeat the process all over again using the same oil and cider vinegar but a fresh batch of herbs.

The same process can be followed using 30 g (1 oz) of dried herbs to half a litre (1 pint) of oil and a tablespoon of cider vinegar. Artificial heat can be used instead of sunlight and at a pinch I do use it during the winter, but the results are not quite as good as by the natural method. Place the jar in a pan of freshly boiled water and try to keep it just below the boil for two hours. This is more difficult than it sounds. You will need to top up the water from time to time and repeat the process daily for two weeks, which is rather tedious. Once the oil smells strong enough to you strain it and rebottle it in a clean dark glass jar. Sticking your nose into the jar and sniffing is not really a fair trial. Treat it like perfume and rub a drop on the pulse point of your wrist. Leave it to sink in and then smell it to see if it is strong enough for your requirements.

Wine maceration usually calls for a handful of fresh herbs or 30 g (1 oz) of dried herbs to a litre (1¾ pints) of either white or red wine. Dried seeds can be successfully used but first bruise them well in a pestle and mortar. Follow the same procedure as for essential oils but macerate for three days only, using the sunlight method. Strain, wash out the bottle, rebottle and cork firmly. White wine is better for fair skins and is a diuretic if taken internally; red wine is better for darker, greasier skins, because being rich in tannin it makes a good astringent. Marie Czetwertynoska, who was the mistress of Alexander I of Russia, used wine with enthusiasm on her skin – she actually bathed in Málaga wine daily. It was then bottled and sold to the unsuspecting. You may plump for moderation, or your purse may do it for you, and decide to use a herbal wine maceration only for a face toner. Use your own discretion as to whether white or red wine would be best for you externally.

Any herbal wine maceration taken internally in moderation is bound to be good for you all over.

The ideal vinegar to use for a *vinegar maceration* is cider vinegar. Wine vinegars are acceptable but malt and white vinegar are far too harsh and smell too strong. Neither should ever be used for cosmetic purposes, not even for hair rinses, unless you want to smell like a fish and chip shop. Cider vinegar will help to restore the acid mantle your skin desperately needs, which is constantly being stripped off by detergents, astringents containing alcohol and by alkaline soaps. It is also particularly good for helping soften rough, flaky skin and for soothing itchy skin. It makes good douches and, used as a hair rinse, not only makes your hair glossy but helps get rid of dandruff without leaving any lingering unpleasant smells. Various herbs can be macerated in both cider and wine vinegars depending on the effect you want to achieve and these herbs are named throughout the ensuing chapters. Use the same process and the same quantities of dried and fresh herbs for a vinegar maceration as for a wine one. Store the vinegar in a dark glass bottle and stopper firmly. Vinegar macerations are ideal for herbs which contain valuable gums and balsamic resins which stubbornly refuse to dissolve in water.

Alcoholic macerations can be made with cheap surgical spirit but I would recommend these only for blistered and tired feet. The rest of the body is too delicate to be dabbed with raw spirit. Vodka, gin and brandy make suitable if expensive alternatives. The comforting thing about these alcohol macerations – or 'tinctures' as they are often called – is that they need only be used very sparingly. Powdered herbs in this instance are more effective than shredded, dried or fresh ones. Use the same quantities and follow the same process as for wine and vinegar macerations, standing the mixture for two weeks in the sunlight. Strain out the powdered herbs through a coffee filter paper and store the tincture in a dark glass bottle very tightly stoppered to prevent evaporation.

Green mulches for external use can be made simply by liquidizing the herb with just enough water to cover the leaves or flowers. Thickened with oatmeal or fuller's earth these make effective if messy face masks. Some herbalists make drinks by the same method but they are almost unpalatable and extremely strong. A dose of watercress drunk like this, for example, would feel as if it were burning your insides out. I would not recommend them.

Essences are simply a small amount of the essential oil of a herb dissolved in a larger quantity of alcohol or vinegar. Use 30 ml (1 fl oz) of essential oil to a litre (1¾ pints) of alcohol. This is an ideal way of making up *herbal waters* as all you then have to do is add a teaspoon of the appropriate essence to half a litre (1 pint) of pure mineral water. Cap the bottle and shake vigorously. Using this method makes herbal and flower waters quite inexpensive and encourages you to use them lavishly. Should your extravagant use of them make you feel guilty, placate yourself with the thought that Saladin had all the walls and floors of the temple in Jerusalem washed with pure rose water before he entered the city in 1187.

Compresses

Some Indian restaurants still follow the custom of offering steaming flannels sprinkled with rose water for you to wipe your hands at the end of a meal. This is really just a modified version of a compress which is a towel or flannel dipped into a warm (not scalding) infusion or decoction, lightly wrung out and applied to the affected area. These are particularly good used alternatively warm and cold to stimulate the circulation of blood in the face or to relieve aching shoulder muscles and legs. Instructions for the legs and shoulders are exactly the same as those which follow for the face, but you may need to use small towels instead of flannels to cover the appropriate area.

Make sure your skin is scrupulously clean and start with a flannel dipped in the warm infusion and lightly wrung out.

Lay it over the face, leaving a gap round your nose so you can breathe. As soon as your face feels warm under the compress, which will be in about thirty seconds, remove the flannel and apply the other flannel dipped in the cold infusion for ten seconds only. Repeat this process four times finishing with the cold compress. This treatment creates a layer of humidity over the skin which acts as a natural moisturizer and is particularly good for dry skin. However, it is not to be used by people with extremely dry flaky skin or thread veins for reasons which are fully explained under the section on thread veins (p. 181).

Cold compresses soothe puffiness, bruising and swelling and reduce large pores. They should never be icy, merely cool, and can be left on the face for up to ten minutes. People with particularly dry skin should massage a few drops of almond oil into it before beginning the treatment.

Syrups

Syrups are best made with honey not sugar. Although many of the old herbals do specify sugar this was because sugar had, since Roman times, been regarded as a medicine rather than as a simple sweetener for culinary use. Consequently, it was included in many comfits to soothe sore throats and in tonics to build up puny children. By Elizabethan times it had become fashionable to use it in household cookery but as it cost a shilling a pound (a day's wages for an artisan) only the very rich could afford it. Consequently, they were the ones who suffered most from blackened rotting teeth.

Sugar gives you nothing but empty calories and, used in syrup-making, it tends to be somewhat difficult to control because it has an annoying habit of turning to caramel as soon as you take your eyes off it. Honey is much easier to use and the ancients considered it one of the foods of the gods. It contains various forms of sugar that are easy to digest, as well as valuable mineral salts and formic acid, which is the bees' own chemical additive that ensures the honey against spoilage and gives it antibacterial qualities. Knights hurt in battle used to have honey poured into their wounds to ensure they would not go septic and to speed up the healing process. Honey is also hydroscopic, that is it has the capacity to attract and hold moisture in the skin so it is helpful for restoring the elasticity in dry ageing skin.

Interestingly, honey contains not only its own sterling qualities but those of the flowers on which the bees have fed. So the famous thyme honey of Greece disinfects the throat and lungs; heather honey helps the urinary system; lime blossom honey is soothing; rosemary honey is stimulating, and clover and orange blossom honey are particularly good for coughs and for soothing sore throats. So sweeten your herbal teas with a honey that will heighten their flavour and underline their effect.

To make a herbal syrup first make a double-strength infusion or decoction in the usual way. Let it brew until it is cold, then strain it, weigh it and pour it in an enamel saucepan before stirring in twice its weight in honey. Thicken slowly over a low heat, stirring gently until the mixture turns syrupy. You may need to skim off scum from time to time. Pot in sterilized jam jars, label and cover tightly. Herbal syrups, apart from making useful and flavoursome spreads and sweeteners, can be added to bath water and to face masks (see section on face masks and on bathing).

Poultices

Poultices may sound old-fashioned but they do have their cosmetic uses and are particularly effective applied to some patches of the body which harbour impurities such as boils and stubborn blackheads. The local application of a poultice has an added bonus as often it ensures that the skin does not get infected in the same area again, at least for some time. So if you are prone to spots in one particular area, first try cleansing your system internally with a fruit and vegetable diet, drink plenty of water and then use poultices externally. The results of such an internal cleansing can be felt after a week, but will not be seen for at least three weeks. Do not be alarmed if your skin gets worse before it gets better with such a cleansing diet.

This condition will only last for four or five days. Poultices may be applied two to three times daily until the area being treated has healed, although for minor eruptions once daily is usually sufficient.

Hot poultices can be made easily by steeping whole fresh leaves in newly boiled water until they are soft. These are then strained, squeezed very gently by hand and applied to the affected area. Speed is essential if you are to derive the full benefit of a poultice but take care not to scald yourself. *Charcoal* poultices are particularly good for really cleansing the skin deeply and drawing out impurities and so are very helpful in the treatment of pustular acne. First, make your own charcoal by toasting three slices of wholemeal bread until they are literally burnt to a cinder. Pound up the charcoal toast to a fine powder in a mortar. Finely grate a couple of scrubbed carrots or a turnip, retaining all their juices. Mix enough, juice and all, into the charcoal to make a thick paste. Spread this directly on to the skin and stay very still for twenty minutes so that it does not start sliding off. Palm off the mask and sluice the face with plenty of barely warm water.

Herbal poultice squares I have so called because I start by spreading a big square of clean lint or gauze on to a large plate. Put the plate on top of a saucepan of simmering water so that most of the underside is heated. Have a quadruple-strength unstrained decoction or infusion of your choice simmering in an enamel saucepan (15 g ($\frac{1}{2}$ oz)) of dried herb to a quarter of a litre ($\frac{1}{2}$ pint) of water should be ample) and slowly add enough coarse slippery elm powder to form a paste. This can usually be obtained from the larger health food shops or from a herbalist. Sprinkle it in with one hand and stir vigorously with the spoon in your other hand. Spread this poultice on to half the fluffy side of the lint but do not take it out to the extreme edge otherwise it will squelch out when you use it. Fold over half the lint so that the poultice is now half a square, pinch the damp edges together and apply the smooth side of the lint gently to the affected part. Once the poultice cools you can reheat it by returning it to the plate still resting over the simmering water. Cover it with another plate. Reheat. Reapply. Do not do this more than twice as the poultice gets weaker every time you use it. Again, remember to test the heat of the poultice with your finger before applying it.

Storing Herbal Preparations

If you mean to drink infusions or decoctions do so immediately. Most of them taste better hot than cold anyway. As with compresses they may safely be kept in a linen-covered glass jar in the fridge for three days. If you put a non-porous cover on this will speed up the fermentation, in which case the mixture should not be kept for longer than a day. If you cannot use the dregs do not pour them down the sink. Your compost heap or the plants in your house and garden will enjoy them much more.

Anything made with alcohol or vinegar will keep for well over a year if stored in sterilized glass jars or bottles which are firmly covered, but do remember that any herbal mixture, no matter how effectively dried or preserved, will grow less effective with age. This is why I advise you to throw out the residue of your dried herbs once they have passed their first birthday. The same is true of vinegar macerations, although their efficacy will usually continue for up to eighteen months. Alcoholic macerations will keep for at least five years.

Because honey is such a good preservative, syrups made with honey should last indefinitely, providing they are always poured into sterilized jars which are kept tightly covered, preferably with a vacuum seal. Essential oils will keep indefinitely stored in small sterilized amber or green bottles. Once the oil gets half-used transfer it to a bottle which is sterilized and smaller still – the elimination of large air gaps will preserve the fragrance of the oil longer. All poultices should be freshly made. Do not try and save the lint afterwards. Throw it away.

You will soon be able to tell if any of your herbal preparations have gone off. They will smell odd and sometimes start to turn an ominous murky green, black or bilious yellow, in which case your compost heap will still be grateful for their libations and you can start again.

Sterilizing containers is a fairly simple process. Wash them in soapy water (and wash the screw-on lids if you are using these). Rinse thoroughly under running warm water. Soak the lids in a diluted mixture of one tablespoon of cider vinegar to a litre (1¾ pints) of water. Put the jars and bottles in a big deep saucepan of water, letting the water run into their insides to sink them. Bring the water to simmering point slowly – 88°C (190°F) – cover and simmer for twenty minutes. Make sure the water does not reach a rapid boil, which will only make the containers crack and knock against each other. Allow the water to cool. Drain the bottles and the caps and place them upside down on a clean tea towel to dry out naturally. Once they have done so screw on the caps and plug any uncapped bottles with wads of cotton wool. When you come to use them you may want to close them with corks, in which case the corks should first be softened and sterilized in diluted vinegar.

Patch Tests

It has been proved that some people are allergic even to water; everything and anything can cause an allergic reaction in someone. In my own experience, while developing and testing my company's range of cosmetic products, I have discovered people who are allergic to innocuous ingredients such as lanolin, henna, glycerine and plant oils – ingredients which have been used safely and effectively by most people for thousands of years. Even herbs, like all medicines, may be potentially dangerous to anyone who suffers from allergies. I am not concerned about synthetic chemical reactions as all the ingredients in this book are of natural origin.

If the ingredients listed in this book are not used properly, if they are taken in excess, used for too long a time, used stale when it has been specifically stated they should be fresh, or taken internally when recommended for external use, they may cause an allergic reaction. I have been careful to point out any herb which may provoke such a reaction and to recommend its exact dosage, processing and specific use. For people who are prone to such sensitivity it is advisable to test some of the more concentrated herbal preparations and some of the raw materials used in this book. To do this simply rub a little of the item you are testing into the pulse point on your wrist, into the crook of your elbow or into the dimple behind your ear. Use enough to cover an area about 2 cm ($\frac{3}{4}$ in.) in diameter. If you are testing something that won't rub into the skin, make a paste of it by pounding it up with a little water. Let the paste dry out and then cover the area with a loose plaster. Leave the patch untouched for twenty-four hours. If the skin feels perfectly comfortable and shows no sign of allergic reaction then you may go ahead and use that ingredient.

For your guidance I list in Appendix I (p. 231) ingredients which I have found from my own experience cause more allergic reactions than others.

Chapter 2

Skin Care

Skin is a complex natural miracle which does far more than merely cover your bones and contain your internal organs. It acts as a protective barrier against the harmful substances which are constantly bombarding it from the outside. Pollution, central heating and some of the components of cosmetics are among the most recent man-made ones.

The epidermis (the outer layer you can actually see) is dead and is made up of flattened cells which are knitted together to form a resilient waterproof surface. This surface is always being rubbed, washed and scaled away. The epidermis is backed by an invisible inner layer (the dermis), which is constantly producing new cells. These journey up to the skin's surface and eventually die and are shed, so that there is a continuous renewal process from the inside out. In fact, a complete renewal takes place over a period of some seven years. This is well worth remembering, because it means no matter what havoc has been wreaked on your skin over the years it is never too late to turn over a new leaf and begin to reap the rewards of a newly cherished skin. No skin is beyond redemption or too old for improvement.

There is a connective layer of collagen fibres between the two layers and when this breaks down or loses its elasticity wrinkles set in. Sweat glands regulate the body's temperature and push out internal waste through the skin. The dermis houses oil glands known as *sebaceous glands*. These exude a fatty substance called *sebum* which lubricates and protects the skin. Unfortunately, very few people are blessed with well-regulated sebaceous glands. Since these are influenced by hormones, sebum production begins in puberty and sometimes runs riot (hence the appearance of teenage acne). The activity of the sebaceous glands tends to lessen in middle age, which is one of the reasons why your skin generally gets progressively drier as you grow older. Dry skin is extremely common. Ninety per cent of women are believed to fall into the dry or combination skin category. The directions for making up a basic cream or lotion on pp. 57–8 suggest lanolin, beeswax or cocoa butter as emollients and emulsifying agents. Lanolin oil very closely resembles our own sebum and its use is particularly advisable for skin that is parchment-fine and producing very little of its own sebum.

Constipation can cause blemishes, which is why it is important to establish regular elimination habits, by which I do not mean the hospital norm which insists you 'move your bowels', as they threateningly put it, at least once a day. Establish your own natural pattern and if you do suffer from chronic constipation the most important thing is to try not to worry about it as this will only make it worse. I have found the following remedies all work. Don't use them all at once, obviously! Try one at a time and stay with the one that suits you until you are back to normal again. Drink at least four pints of water daily. Adulterated water – tea, coffee and fruit juice – does not count. Drinking water is not only a good remedy for eliminating constipation, it also helps to keep the skin clear and healthy and encourages sparkling eyes and sweet breath, so try and make it part of your daily routine. Other remedies for constipation include a tablespoon of cider vinegar sweetened with a teaspoon of honey or black strap molasses dissolved in a big mug of hot water first thing in the morning; a big bowl of strawberries daily; two to three teaspoons of violet syrup daily (see p. 210); four to five cups of marshmallow tea drunk at regular intervals throughout the day, or a double-strength decoction of dandelion leaves, one wineglassful to be taken before meals. All of these remedies will help to flush out the toxins in your body which, if left to stagnate, struggle up to the skin's surface and appear as blemishes, poor pasty skin colour or dark circles under the eyes.

The skin is a two-way street. Not only can it push things

out, it can also absorb things. Substances fed into the body can appear in the skin and substances fed into the skin can appear in the body. This is why it is important to put on your skin only things that you would be prepared to eat or drink. That may well make you blanch and throw out your cosmetics and aftershaves because you do not know what is in them. It has been proved that indelible dyes which are still used in some lipsticks are photosensitive and can cause cracking, drying and peeling. Ammonium sulphide which appears in some deodorants and other cosmetics can make some people react with rashes, swellings and cracked skin. The alcohol in aftershaves can irritate and dry out the skin. Certain preservatives in cosmetics can also cause allergic reactions. These substances are unpleasant enough on the skin; the thought of their effects on one's insides is not appealing. Happily the United States Food and Drug Administration is now very stringent about the open declaration of cosmetic ingredients on the packaging and the European Economic Community is soon to follow suit. Japan has already established strict regulations in this field. But it is up to you to read about the ingredients before you buy them.

It is as well to remember that not so very long ago science viewed skin merely as an excreting 'envelope' which protected the internal organs from external invasion. The skin's need to breathe and its vulnerability to surface toxicants is a relatively new concept. Blood tests can reveal the presence of toxic materials absorbed into the blood stream through the skin. Witches were able to poison people or to get high by rubbing into the skin various ointments which contained extracts from such herbs as henbane, deadly nightshade, hemlock, monkshood and sea holly, which proves the permeability of the skin. It works the other way round as well, of course. You can influence the skin and hair from the inside of the body. For example, if you take an aspirin 25 per cent of it appears in the hair within nine hours and it takes nineteen days for its presence to be completely eradicated. The prolonged ingestion of aspirin will eventually weaken the structure of the hair.

So, what you feed your skin from the inside is of fundamental importance. Nutrition is still a young science: much has yet to be established, and meanwhile we are deluged with facts which often leave us confused and undecided. Natural vitamins versus synthetic ones? Minerals, bran, polyunsaturated oils, vegetarianism? Everyone seems to have their favourite hobby-horse. Chapter 7 is full of advice about diet. Sufficient to say here that you should keep your diet high in protein and raw vegetables and fruit and remember my previous advice about water. Also, try to eat at least half your daily requirements raw to ensure that you are not boiling away valuable minerals and vitamins.

Vitamins

There are abundant herbal sources of vitamins which are cheap and easily available if you take the trouble to grow them or find them yourself. Vitamin A is good for nearly every part of you – hair, skin, nails, teeth and eyes. Lack of it causes scaliness, large pores, dry rough skin and blemishes as well as scalp abscesses and loss of hair. However, you are extremely unlikely to be short of vitamin A: this is one of the few vitamins you can overdose yourself with as it is not water-soluble – it needs fats to be properly used by the body. Dandelion leaves, watercress and parsley are particularly rich in vitamin A.

The vitamin B complex is essential for healthy skin and hair. It also helps fatigue, insomnia, checks irritability and helps to clear up acne and eczema. It is available in liver, wheatgerm, brewer's yeast, brown rice, tuna and halibut, yoghurt and black molasses.

Vitamin C is a must for those who eat a high-protein diet, because the more protein you eat the more vitamin C your body requires. The average person needs 60 mg a day although individual needs can range quite widely. Smokers, for example, need more because each cigarette burns up 25 mg. Bleeding gums and easily bruised muscles can be prevented by vitamin C, which speeds up the healing process, prevents fatigue, helps destroy virus infections, bacteria and poisons and can sometimes help skin abnormalities which are the result of allergies. Good sources of vitamin C are rosehips, citrus fruits, blackcurrants, strawberries, cabbage, cauliflower and potatoes.

The skin produces its own vitamin D when it is exposed to the sun but it is easily destroyed by alkaline soaps. The main foods that provide vitamin D are herrings, mackerel, butter, margarine and cheese. Lack of this vitamin causes tooth decay and bone deformation. Vitamin E is found in corn oil, cotton oil, ground nut oil, soya bean oil, sunflower seed oil and, of course, in wheatgerm and wheatgerm oil. Not only does it protect your herbal creams against oxidation (see p. 56), it also protects all the cells in your body against ageing by oxidation. Taken internally it prevents unsightly liver spots and varicose veins, helps muscle tone generally and promotes the circulation. Taken externally vitamin E helps to heal scars, though some dermatologists also believe it thins the skin while doing so. I have never found this to be the case in my own experiments. Indeed, wheatgerm oil, in particular, seems to make tired skin look fresher and more resilient.

Minerals

Minerals are another comparatively uncharted territory in nutritional terms. A supply of adequate and correctly balanced mineral salts is believed to retard old age (although controversy about this still rages) and to help resist illness. Calcium, coupled with vitamin C, forms collagen fibres which support the skin, keeping it firm and resilient and preventing stretch marks and wrinkles. Linked with one-and-a-half times its weight of phosphorus it helps to build healthy bones and teeth. It is also a natural tranquillizer. There are many excellent herbal sources of calcium: arrowroot, chamomile, chives, coltsfoot, dandelion leaves and root, horsetail, meadowsweet, nettle, pimpernel, sorrel and rest harrow. The calcium content of a plant is radically reduced by the use of artificial fertilizers – generally the darker the leaf the more calcium it contains.

Without phosphorus the body cannot adequately or

efficiently turn the B complex vitamins into energy: it helps lecithin's action as a fat-dissolving agent. Calamus, chickweed, garlic, liquorice root, marigolds, meadowsweet, sorrel and caraway seeds are all excellent herbal sources of phosphorus.

Iron is essential for the blood and the liver. Growing children need lots of it, so do women during pregnancy, during menstruation and after the menopause. Half a cupful of parsley contains more iron than a quarter of a pound of liver! Other rich herbal sources of iron are burdock root, meadowsweet, mullein leaves, rest harrow, nettles, strawberry leaves and

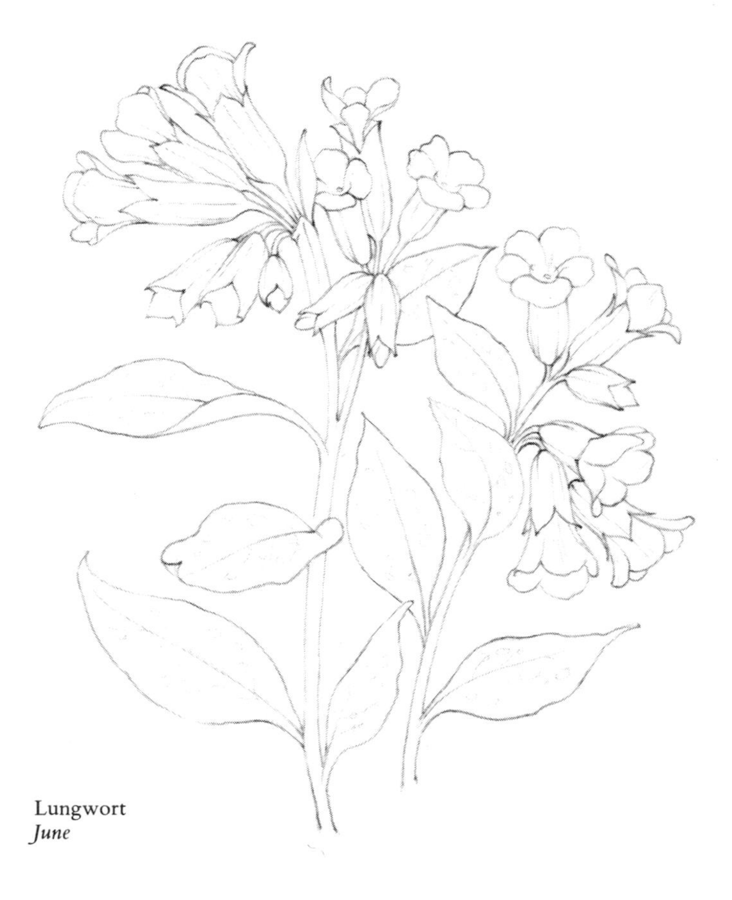

Lungwort
June

dock. Iron cannot function properly to help the body without an adequate supply of copper – lack of copper can result in greying hair, heart disorders and general nervousness. Herbal sources of copper are burdock root, parsley, nettles, watercress and yellow dock.

Iodine is needed by the scavenger cells of our bodies called *phagocytes*, to do their excellent and very necessary work efficiently. Herbal sources of iodine include bladderwrack, dulse, kelp and garlic.

Silicon promotes the growth of protein (your hair and nails) and helps to keep your skin from becoming flabby as well as contributing towards good eyesight. The eyes contain about twenty times more silicon than the muscles and there is about 20 per cent less silicon in older people's skin than in young people's. A high percentage of silicon is available in horsetail, comfrey, dandelion, nettles, hound's tongue and lungwort. The importance of another mineral, magnesium, is discussed on p. 194.

Skin Types

Do you know what your skin type is?

Dry Skin

Dry skin feels thin and delicate and sometimes you cannot see any pores in it at all. It feels parched and stretched tight across the bones after washing, and has a tendency to develop myriads of tiny lines around the eyes which soon turn into full-blown wrinkles if neglected. It may also appear flaky in patches and show tiny thread veins. Dry skin can be washed with soap and water, providing the soap is a glycerine or pure castile one, preferably one you have concocted yourself (see the soap section later in the chapter). Very thin delicate skin may be better off with nut or oatmeal washes and pores should never be clogged with anything containing alcohol – a diluted herbal water or, better still, a herbal milk is preferable. The one essential for this skin type is to moisturize and moisturize again but never with a rich oily cream, which only makes the skin so lazy that it stops producing its own sebum altogether. Men who shave with a blade should wash first with a herbal soap, sluice the soap away with lots of water and apply a moisturizer to the still damp skin. They should then apply shaving foam or soap, leaving it to soften and wet the beard for two or three minutes before beginning the long scrape. This advice also applies to women who shave their legs. Under no circumstances should men use a cologne or aftershave on the face afterwards. If they must use something, a spicy diluted herbal water should suffice and will not rob the skin of its sorely needed moisture (see Chapter 4). They should then use a moisturizer liberally on a still damp skin. (Of course, freshly shaved legs should also be protected by at least two applications of a light body lotion.)

Oily Skin

Oily skin shines with grease, looks thick and coarse and often has enlarged pores and blackheads. It looks toneless and muddy in colour. All this may sound discouraging but in fact its one big bonus is that it ages well, showing fewer wrinkles and lines than dry skin. Oily skin tends to attract pollutants like a magnet, so it should be thoroughly cleansed three times a day if possible with any soap other than superfatted or cocoa butter ones which tend to leave a residue on this skin type. Oily skin needs toning but, contrary to popular belief, alcohol astringents only dehydrate the skin, causing dry patches, and further coarsen the texture of the skin. Use diluted herbal vinegars for refining the pores and don't forget to moisturize with a light non-greasy cream, spreading it thickly over a still damp skin. Exfoliant masks are very important for this skin type. Not only do they help unclog blocked pores but they accelerate the sloughing off of the debris of dead cells which causes the skin to look coarse and leathery. Men should never use a facial steam and exfoliant mask before shaving. Make it a bed-time treat instead.

Combination Skin

Combination skin is usually a mixture of the two skin types above: an oily panel runs down the centre of the face and across the forehead while the cheeks remain dry and sometimes flaky. Unfortunately, combination skins are very common. They are also the most trouble to look after because they have to be treated as two different skins, as indeed they are. It is quite usual for men to have combination skin as a result of shaving.

Old-looking Skin

Old-looking skin may not necessarily be anything to do with years; it may simply be the result of neglect. It is often thin, extremely sensitive and looks crepey, saggy, sometimes with enlarged pores and a coarse texture. It may be pasty white or sallow in colour. This type of skin needs special repair and care. Nourish it with the right balance of raw and protein-rich foods internally (cod liver oil tablets work wonders) and cherish it with a gentle hand and lots of vitamin-rich oils and honey externally. If the skin is thin it should never be subjected to exfoliation. Open pores can be refined with lemon juice, diluted herbal wine, buttermilk and orange flower water, all of which will also help to lift sallowness out of the skin.

Normal Skin

I sometimes wonder if there is such a thing. Ideally it should be unblemished, satin-smooth, supple and resilient to the touch, and it has an inner translucency which makes it glow. If you are one of the lucky few who own such a miracle of nature be thankful and look after it. Complacency will not help it stay that way. Twice-daily washing with a pure castile herbal soap, toning with a flower or herbal water and moisturizing thoroughly over a damp skin will preserve your good fortune. If the skin starts to look dull an exfoliant mask may prove necessary to remove the debris which is masking that inner glow. All this advice applies to black skin too, although generally black skin seems to age more slowly than its white counterpart for various environmental and genetic reasons: black people, for example, are usually less inclined to subject themselves to the ravages of sunbathing.

No matter what your skin type the first step towards its improvement is thorough cleansing. This is much more than a cosmetic consideration and is just as important for men as for women. The body's oils and waste are excreted on to the surface of the skin and are joined there by external atmospheric pollution. This motley assortment of decomposed cells, sebum, sweat, bacteria and pollutants will soon block the pores if it is not carefully and regularly removed. A quick swish of water and soap will not do. Indeed, it may further aggravate your facial debris by adding residual soap to it and drawing precious moisture from the cells which may already be desiccated.

Cleansing

Soap seems to lie at the centre of the great skin care debate so let me, if you will forgive the pun, begin by dishing the dirt. Some experts are utterly opposed to washing with soap at all, believing there are better non-alkaline ways of cleansing the skin. The whole concept of acid–alkaline balance needs explanation. Normal healthy skin and hair are slightly acidic and this acidity comes from the skin's secretions (particularly from the sebaceous glands). These form the skin's acid mantle which protects and lubricates the skin. The pH (hydrogen potential) factor in any soap, shampoo or cosmetic product is the relative degree of acidity or alkalinity in that product. Some companies make soaps, shampoos and cleansers with a pH that corresponds to the acid mantle, but this ignores the fact that the pH of the skin varies from person to person and at different times in the same parts of the same person. When the pH is artificially altered the body will, unassisted, return to its usual pH within a few hours. The pH of the skin is measured on a scale from 0 to 14 and is generally about 5·5. A skin registering between 5·4 and 6·2 shows a mildly acid condition which means it's at its peak, well-protected from infection by its acid mantle because bacteria which is constantly settling on the skin cannot live on an acid surface. A pH of 6·2 to 7 means the skin does not have enough acid and, as it is a bit alkaline, will tend to be more prone to infection. If the pH is below 5·4 the skin will be too acid and feel extremely sensitive. However, soap's alkalinity is one of the very things that enables it to cleanse so thoroughly and I don't think you can beat the lovely fresh feeling of a soap and water wash followed by a rinse with cider vinegar, which will help to correct the pH balance of your skin.

For centuries now soap has been made from water, sodium salts, fatty acids and various oils. Modern detergent soaps are really soapless because chemicals have taken the place of the various natural ingredients, but all soaps carry out the same task of loosening dead skin cells, degreasing the skin and dislodging dirt, so that the whole mess can be rinsed away with water. Castile soap made with olive oil or a glycerine soap are the ones I recommend. If you take the trouble to make your own soap, the glycerine in the fats and oils you use is retained. In commercial products it is removed and sold separately, although you can buy commercial glycerine-based soaps, some of which are very good. People with delicate flaky skin usually benefit from the use of such a soap.

Simple Herbal Soapmaking

Making your own soap from scratch requires the use of caustic soda which can burn unprotected skin horribly. Its fumes can scar the lungs and hurt the eyes so I suggest you start one step further along and avoid these dangers.

Buy some bars of castile soap and grate them or, alternatively, buy some castile soap flakes. Take 120 g (4 oz) of dried or four heaped handfuls of fresh herbs or flowers suitable for your skin type (see p. 63) and cover with a cup of water. If you are using a fresh herb pound it to a thick mulch with your pestle and mortar before covering it with the water. Dried herbs need no preliminary preparation. Simmer the whole mixture very gently indeed for ten minutes, remembering to cover tightly. Leave to infuse overnight. Strain through coffee filter paper and add this liquid to the shaved soap. You can use anything between 120 g (4 oz) and half a kilo (1 lb). The more soap you add the more solid your end product will be.

Melt down the soap over a gentle heat in an enamel pot, stirring vigorously with a wooden spoon or a balloon whisk so that the herbal liquid is well amalgamated. Let the mixture cool a little and add a few drops of an appropriate essential oil to give the soap some fragrance. Then pour the soap into greased moulds or into a small wet wooden box lined with a wet cotton cloth. Leave the soap to dry. This may take four hours or it may take as much as a week, depending on how much mucilage and tannin the herb you used contained. Unmould the soap, and cut it up into bars. Wrap it in greaseproof paper and let it age with dignity in your airing cupboard for at least a month. The longer you leave it (within reason) the nicer it will smell and meanwhile it will scent all your linen and towels.

The consistency of your final product will depend on the herbs you have chosen. Herbs with a lot of mucilage, such as houseleek, comfrey and marshmallow, produce softer soap and generally require more water. The manufacturer's original formulation for castile soap – and it does vary quite widely – will also determine the consistency of your soap. So don't be afraid to experiment, then when you attain perfection remember to make careful notes about how you did it (where you purchased your castile flakes, what herb you used and at what time of year you picked it).

You can replace half the soap with honey in the melting stage if you have a very sensitive or crepey skin or replace a quarter of the soap with anhydrous lanolin if you have a very parched skin. Melt the lanolin separately first in a double boiler and then add it to the herbal decoction and the melted castile soap in a thin stream, beating hard all the time. If using solid honey treat it in the same way, though there is no need to take the trouble to melt liquid honey. You can also add a few teaspoons of oil for very dry skin.

Houseleek and Honey Soap (for dry, sensitive skins)

60 g (2 oz) marshmallow leaves

60 g (2 oz) houseleek

2 cups water

120 g (4 oz) honey

270 g (9 oz) castile soap

Follow directions above.

Oatmeal and Lavender Soap (for greasy skins)

60 g (2 oz) oatmeal

120 g (4 oz) lavender

1 cup water

270 g (9 oz) castile soap

essential oil of lavender (optional)

Follow directions above, adding the oatmeal only once the soap has melted and the lavender water has been stirred in. If you decide to heighten the fragrance of the soap still further add the lavender oil then. Let the mixture become cool enough to enable you to form the soap into little balls. The gritty oatmeal makes it a good exfoliant.

Lettuce Soap (for normal skins)

120 g (4 oz) shredded lettuce

1 cup water

240 g (9 oz) pulverized almonds

60 g (2 oz) honey

270 g (9 oz) castile soap

essential oil of chamomile (optional)

Follow the directions above, mashing the lettuce in the infusion with a wooden spoon to extract all of its properties. Substitute almond meal for the oatmeal and add the honey at the beginning of the melting process. This soap is particularly nice scented with chamomile oil.

A Delicate Washing-Ball

'Take three ounces of orace [orris root], halfe an ounce of Cypres [bark], two ounces of Calamus Aromaticus [the root of sweet flag], one ounce of Rose leaves, two ounces of Lavender flowers: beat all these together in a mortar, searcing them [sieving them] through a fine Searce, then scrape some Castill sope, and dissolve it with some Rose-water, then incorporate all your powders therewith, by labouring them well in a mortar.'

Ram's Little Dodeon, 1606

I took 'some Castill sope' to mean three quarters of a kilo ($1\frac{1}{2}$ lb) and added half a litre (1 pint) of rose water. I gave up on the Cypres bark as I could not reduce it to the necessary powder either in my mortar or my liquidizer. I used rose petals instead of leaves. The result was a sweet-smelling, slightly gritty soap ball which toned up the skin very effectively. I noticed the soap turned slightly brown after a while but it kept its interesting fragrance.

Balles for the Face

'Take great Allecant reusons [raisins] a quarter of a pounde, stone them but wash them not and beat them in a mortar very fine, take as many almonds, not jordans, but of the common sort and blanck [blanche] them and dry them in a cloth well and beate them in a stone mortar also very fine, when you have done this to them bothe, mingle them bothe together and beate them againe, and put to it half a pound of browne leavened bread, wheaten bread, and beate them altogether and mingle them well together and then take it and make it in little balles and then wash your face at night with one of them in rayne water. If you will have this only to wash your hands, put in a little Venice soape but put none of that in for youre face.'

Mary Fairfax, *Still-Room Book*, 1632

I used plump stoned raisins, skinned almonds and wholemeal bread, and had to restrain myself from eating it. I quartered the

Orris Root
October

original quantity as the mixture is entirely organic and if not used up quickly tends to sprout robust penicillin mould. The smell was superb. It reminded me of Christmas. The balls soon fall apart in your hand and turn into a very effective scrub. Particularly good for dry dingy skin in need of a spring clean.

How to Wash your Face

Having made your soap learn to use it properly. Begin by splashing your face with lots of warm water. Then work up a good lather in your hands from a bar of herbal soap appropriate for your skin type. Spread this on your face and gently massage upwards and outwards, skimming lightly around the eyes and paying special attention to the nose and chin. Now sluice the soap off with lots of warm water. Run a basin of fresh, barely tepid water and add a tablespoon of cider vinegar to it. This will help restore the acid mantle your skin so badly needs to fend off bacteria and infection for its protection. Splash at least twenty handfuls of this rinse on to your face. Palm your skin dry, that is, pat away the water using the palms of your hands, leaving it slightly damp so that you can apply a moisturizer. This method of drying does not roughen the skin cells as an abrasive towel does and, much more importantly it leaves some of the water on the skin's surface to moisturize it and to be held there by a cling film of moisturizer.

Never use large quantities of cold water as a rinse. This will only aggravate sensitive skin and thread veins and make the sebaceous glands pump out oil even harder after their initial cold shock. You can, if you like, spray your face with a plant mister containing one of the mineral waters or herbal vinegar or wine mixes suitable for your skin type (see p. 63). Leave this untouched on the skin for a few minutes, then apply a layer of moisturizer over it.

For those still not totally convinced by the argument in favour of soap, soapwort is an excellent herbal substitute which can be used on any skin type. The root yields a lot of mucilage which, mixed with water, resembles soap in solution. The saponin in it is the cleansing agent. Boil up 30 g (1 oz) of the shredded root in a litre (1¾ pints) of water in a covered pot and simmer for twenty minutes. Cool, strain and use the decoction as a shampoo for the hair or the skin. Soapwort is particularly good for cleansing itchy, chapped skin. Fumitory and marshmallow were also celebrated for their cleansing powers and were extensively used in washballs but are not quite as effective as soapwort.

Cleansing Creams and Lotions

Skin can also be cleansed by cleansing creams and lotions which liquefy on the skin (because of its warmth) and loosen and suspend the debris there. Having been tissued away they leave a greasy residue which must be removed with a toner. Omitting the second step is as bad as not cleansing the skin at all. A cleanser is like the carriage part of the proverbial horse and carriage. Without the horsepower of the toner it is useless.

Nearly all commercial cleansing creams contain mineral oil – the sort of thing which is sometimes sold as baby oil. It should not be used either on you or on babies because it robs your body of the fat-soluble vitamins A, D, E and K. (Remember, the skin is a two-way street and mineral oil quickly passes through the skin into the blood stream dissolving the fat-soluble vitamins on its way and leading to possible vitamin deficiencies.) If you take mineral oil as a laxative it does the same thing – all the fat-soluble vitamins appear in the faeces. It is important to retain as many of your vitamins as possible so I feel mineral oil should never be used by anyone under any circumstances. Use a combination of natural plant and nut oils together with anhydrous lanolin or beeswax, which will act as a solidifier. Using natural oils means your creams will go off more quickly than their synthetic counterparts but then you are probably not planning to make up gallons of cream at a time.

Natural preservatives. Wheatgerm oil will act as an anti-oxidant and stop creams going rank and turning dark brown. Simple tincture of benzoin – a balsamic resin extracted from trees in Java – will lengthen the shelf life of creams and lotions as will tincture of myrrh, a resin used in incense. Use myrrh for oily skins, benzoin for dry, delicate skins. Witchhazel will also help to preserve creams but it is not as effective. As a general rule of thumb, decoctions which have been subjected to a long boiling which kills most bacteria are less likely to make creams go off than infusions. Either way, when adding water to a cream always make sure it has been boiled or purified. Moulds start once the cream is exposed to the air so cut out a little disc from waxed or greaseproof paper or silver foil and lay this on top of the cream as soon as it has been potted. If you really must make up a large batch, keep whatever you are not using in the refrigerator. Try not to let other people use your cream. This may sound inordinately fussy but recent research has revealed that the bacteria passed from one person's skin to another via the use of a communal cream may cause infections.

A lotion is simply a thinned-down version of a cream which contains less of the thickening agents lanolin and beeswax. The beauty of making your own creams is that, depending on what herbs you add to them, they can be made to fulfil all sorts of functions – antiseptic, astringent, soothing or stimulating, drying or hydrating. You can reinforce the action of the herb in its infusion or decoction form by adding the same herb in its essential oil form. Either way, you have the assurance of knowing that you are only including items that are fit to eat and, this being the case, they will certainly be good enough for cherishing your skin.

Lanolin. You will notice that in the Basic Cream Directions which follow you are given the choice of lanolin, beeswax or cocoa butter as your emulsifier. Lanolin is the oil washed from the wool of sheep once they have been sheared and it is rather like the sebum the skin produces as a protective lubricant. It is also an excellent moisturizer as it is capable of attracting moisture from the air. Your chemist will probably offer you two types of lanolin: hydrous and anhydrous. Always use anhydrous lanolin, which is not mixed with extra water, except for the few recipes which specifically require hydrous lanolin, such as cleansing creams. Their purpose is to remove the dirt from your skin in a slurry, not to moisturize it.

Glycerine is another excellent humectant. Very little of the glycerine that is commercially available today is made in the old-fashioned way, using animal bones. Most glycerine is now a product of chemical synthesis and therefore does not involve cruelty to animals. There is some glycerine available which has a vegetable base and it might be worth inquiring about this from the better stocked health food shops. However, I have found it difficult to track down as very few places stock it, although persistent demand may change this.

Benzoin. Two types of benzoin are made: simple tincture of benzoin and compound tincture of benzoin. Always make sure you buy the simple tincture as the compound one is toxic and can be harmful to the skin.

Basic Cream Directions

1 30 g (1 oz) of lanolin or beeswax. You can use both at the same time, varying the proportion, as long as they add up to 30 g in all. Beeswax will give your creams a stiffer, shinier consistency. You can also incorporate cocoa butter, mixing it with either the lanolin or beeswax. Cocoa butter will make your cream feel rich and oily. However, some people are allergic to cocoa butter and a few to lanolin so try a patch test first (see p. 37).

2 120 ml (4 fl oz) of any natural oil. Again, you can use a blend of several as long as they make up this quantity in all. I always use at least 20 ml (⅔ fl oz or 4 tsp) wheatgerm oil as part of my oil selection because of its marvellous healing properties as well as its anti-oxidant capacity. Use only 90 ml (3 fl oz) of oil for a less rich cream.

3 30 ml (1 fl oz or 2 tbsp) of any herb infusion, decoction or flower water.

4 Three to six drops of any essential oil from a herb or flower. This is optional and the number of drops you add will depend on the strength of the essential oil and on how strong you want the cream to smell.

Melt the lanolin and/or beeswax in the top of an enamel double boiler. The use of a double boiler prevents the lanolin from burning – and burnt lanolin smells terrible. Now slowly add the oil a bit at a time, beating with your special cosmetic wooden spoon or a whisk. Do not use a balloon whisk in this instance because it will incorporate too many air bubbles into the cream. Remove the boiler from the stove and slowly add the herbal water, a trickle at a time, still beating constantly. Once it is all incorporated, slow to a steady stir until the cream has cooled to blood heat. Now is the time to add your choice of essential oil. If you add it any earlier the heat of the cream will distort some of the more delicate top notes of oil. This quantity will make about 180 g (6 oz) of cream, so have a large wide-necked opaque sterilized jar standing by and spoon the mixture into it.

A lotion is as easy to make as a cream. It is just a matter of varying the proportion of the ingredients.

Basic Lotion Directions

1 30 g (1 oz) of lanolin or beeswax or a combination of both. Cocoa butter can also be used for a richer, oilier cream. Try a patch test on lanolin or cocoa butter first to make sure you are not allergic to them before beginning.

2 90 ml (3 fl oz) of any natural oil, preferably including 10 ml of wheatgerm oil.

3 60 ml (2 fl oz) of any herbal infusion, decoction or flower water.

4 Three to six drops of essential oil from any herb or flower.

Melt the lanolin and/or beeswax in the top of an enamel double boiler. Add the oil, beating steadily with your cosmetic wooden spoon, then the water which should be added in a slow trickle. Take the boiler off the stove and continue to stir steadily until the lotion has cooled to blood heat. Now add the essential oil. Stir it in thoroughly and decant the lotion into a half-litre (1 pint) bottle. Screw on the cap or cork and shake desultorily until the lotion has entirely cooled. This occasional shaking once every few minutes is necessary to stop the oil and water phases of the lotion separating out while it is warm. Do not forget to label your jars and bottles.

Whether following directions for a cream or a lotion follow these recipes exactly. If after a few attempts you decide you would prefer a thicker or thinner mixture simply vary the amount of emulsifier, oil or water. More lanolin will make the cream thicker and tackier. Less will make it runnier. More cocoa butter will make the cream both thicker and oilier. More water will obviously thin the cream as will more oil, which will also make it greasier.

Variations should not extend to more than 10 g or 20 ml (½ oz) either way or the cream will fail to emulsify. Remember the texture of the cream will also vary depending on which oils and which herbs you use. Ground nut oil will obviously make the cream less slick in consistency than almond oil. Herbs with a lot of mucilage will make the cream feel spongier.

Lemon Verbena Cleanser (for dry and sensitive skins)

Coconut oil and cocoa butter are two of the best natural cleansers for this skin type. Following the directions for a basic cream, substitute cocoa butter for half the lanolin and use hydrous lanolin. Use rose water or an infusion of lemon balm as your herbal water and add essential oil of lemon verbena which marries well with the balm and is both soothing and toning.

Rose Cleanser (for normal and combination skins)

You could not do better than follow the recipe of the Greek physician, Galen, who first invented cleansing cream nearly 1,800 years ago. Following the basic cream directions use hydrous lanolin, almond oil, rose water and essential oil of roses.

Cucumber and Yarrow Cleanser (for oily skins)

Oily skins are better cleansed with a lotion rather than a cream. Liquidize a quarter of a cucumber and strain out the resulting juice through a coffee filter paper. Make a double-strength infusion of yarrow using 30 g (1 oz) of dried yarrow to a cup of water. Strain this. Measure out 30 ml (1 fl oz) of both liquids.

Blend, using corn oil and hydrous lanolin and following the basic directions for a lotion. Add six drops of tincture of myrrh when you add your essential oil, which can either be lavender or rose geranium.

Comfrey and Houseleek Cleanser (for old-looking skins)

Make a decoction of 30 g (1 oz) of finely chopped houseleek leaves by simmering them in a cup of water for twenty minutes in a tightly covered enamel saucepan. Keep covered and allow to cool. Strain and measure out 30 ml (1 fl oz). Follow the basic cream directions using avocado oil and substituting cocoa butter for the lanolin. Once the cream is at blood heat add six drops of essential oil of comfrey and six drops of simple tincture of benzoin.

Deep Cleansing

For an extra thorough cleanse try a facial steam. Oily skin

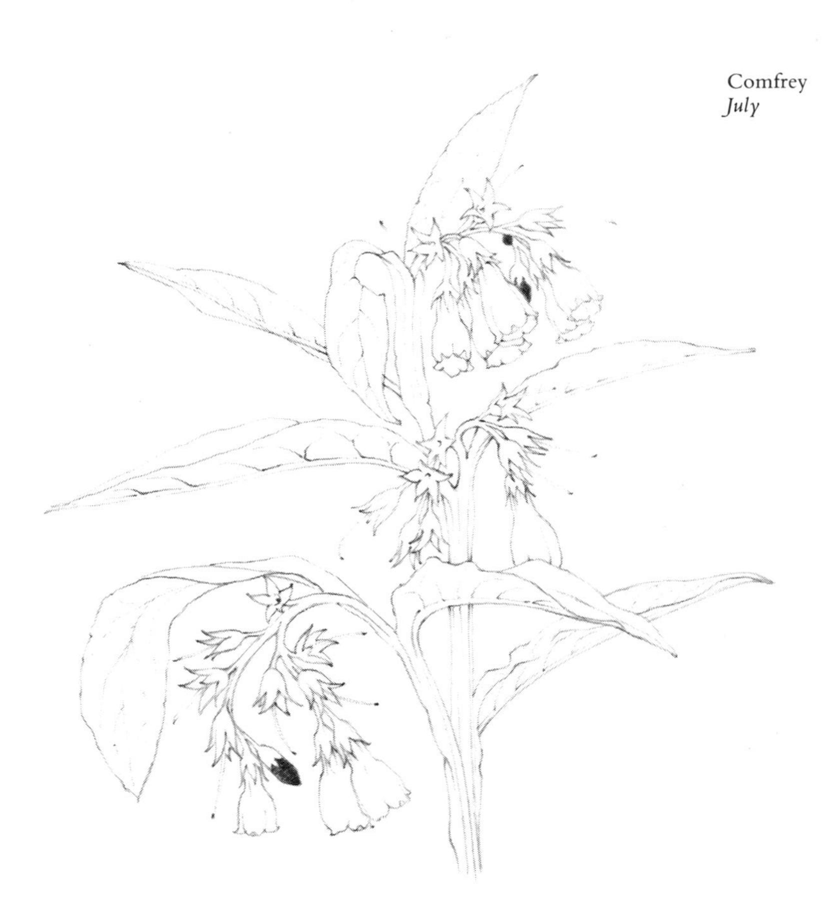

Comfrey
July

types can use this twice a week as well as their normal soap and water routine. Dry, sensitive skin types should try this in place of soap and water once fortnightly. All other skin types can safely use a facial steam once a week in place of soap and water or a cleansing cream.

Directions for a Herbal Steam

Cleanse or wash your face as usual leaving your skin moist. Put two heaped tablespoons of dried herbs or three heaped handfuls of fresh ones in a non-metal basin and pour over 2 litres ($3\frac{1}{2}$ pints) of boiling water. Stir the herbs well into the water with a wooden spoon. Tie your hair back or tuck it into a plastic bath hat. Now hold your face at least 20 cm (8 in.) away from the water and trap the rising steam with a thick towel held over your head and the basin. Keep your eyes closed and let the steam work on your face for at least ten minutes. You can poke your head out for air from time to time if you have to.

People with thin or sensitive skin should hold their faces 45 cm (18 in.) away from the water, and should first moisturize the face with a little diluted herbal vinegar and then immediately massage in half a teaspoon of one of the vitamin E-rich oils. Those who have thread veins should avoid the use of a herbal steam altogether. They should use a warm or cold comfrey compress instead as an occasional aid to deep cleansing. Asthmatics and people who suffer from heart trouble should not use this method of cleansing.

Given these exceptions, a herbal steam is superb for deeply cleansing every pore, as well as increasing the elimination of toxins by raising the perspiration level, increasing circulation and hydrating the skin by adding moisture.

Once the steam is completed strain out the herbs with a nylon sieve and save them for your compost heap. Rinse with the remaining herbal water, then with cool (not cold) water to close the pores, or use a diluted herbal vinegar. Stay inside for about two hours before braving the elements and pollution outside: it takes time for the pores to refine themselves. Any blackheads or whiteheads should be squeezed out gently immediately after the steam with fingertips protected with tissues or cotton wool. A movement in which you gently shift your fingertips round the spot as you squeeze steadily is more effective than squeezing hard from both sides. Be especially conscientious about protecting the pores after removing blemishes. Yarrow, tansy or violet teas, witchhazel or diluted simple tincture of benzoin are all effective pore-refiners.

When using any of the following herbs for your skin type for a facial steam select at least three and mix them in equal quantities. It is quite handy to mix up half a kilo (1 lb) at a time and keep them in a large screw-top jar so that they are readily available. Any of the herbs suitable for your skin type can be used in creams, masks, lotions, aftershaves and hair treatments. I have stated specific herbs and combinations in recipes only because I have found them to be the most effective for their selected task. You may like to experiment by substituting others from your skin type group. Use the leaves of all the herbs listed unless otherwise indicated.

Herbs for Various Skin Types

Oily Skins

comfrey (root, leaves)
fennel (leaves, seeds)
geranium leaves
horsetail
lavender
lupin seeds
marigold (flowers)
nettles
peppermint
sage
yarrow

Use up to two tablespoons of these for a facial steam and add three drops of simple tincture of benzoin to the water.

Dry, Sensitive Skins

borage (leaves, flowers)
houseleek
lady's mantle
marshmallow (leaves, root)
salad burnet
sorrel
pansy (flowers)
parsley
violets (leaves, flowers)

Combination Skins

bay
chamomile (flowers)
comfrey
meadowsweet (flowers)

rosemary
thyme
whole rose petals

Old, Sallow, Crepey Skins

daisies (flowers)
dandelion (leaves)
elderflowers
lemon verbena
liquorice root (decoction)
red clover (leaves, flowers)
tansy (flowers, leaves)

Normal Skins

applemint
comfrey (root, leaves)
cowslip (flowers)
lemon balm
lime flowers
spearmint

A word of warning about cowslips. They can produce in some people a condition known as *primula dermatitis*, a dark scabby eruption which is the result of placing the flower directly on the skin. So by all means use the flower freely in facial steams, teas, food and skin lotions, but never rub it on the skin. This allergy is quite rare but do not let yourself be one of the unlucky few.

All these herbs, with the exception of cowslips, liquorice and any other roots can be used either by themselves or in combination as a green mulch face mask for the appropriate skin types. Seeds, of course, must first be pounded to a powder in a mortar, though they can be used whole in a facial steam. Macerate any dried herbs intended for a mask in a splash of hot water to plump them up before straining and mixing them in.

Masks are particularly effective for clearing up blemishes, refining open pores and coarse skin, nourishing, healing and soothing the skin, absorbing excessive oil, moisturizing or lubricating the skin and for temporarily firming up and tightening the skin as well as exfoliating the epidermis. It is occasionally necessary to do this when too many dead skin cells have accumulated and are not being removed by simple soap and water washing. The dead cells build up, leaving the skin looking dingy and sallow. Men who shave exfoliate every day (except on the unshaven areas like the nose, cheeks and forehead). It may be specially necessary to exfoliate once the skin has reached the tail end of a sun-tan as tanning actually thickens the skin. Pawpaw, pineapple and figs are all superb exfoliants as they contain special protein-digesting enzymes which are capable of softening protein tissue. Pawpaw is certainly the strongest and should be used with care. All these fruits should be mashed and then held in a sieve to allow any excess juice to drain away. I was brought up in Tanzania and we used to tenderize any tough meat by marinading it in mashed pawpaw. So if it tenderizes meat it will certainly make your skin feel softer.

Do not neglect the rest of your body if you are treating yourself to a mask. Dry flaky elbows, knees, heels and throats could all benefit from a mask. This applies just as much to men as to women. Remember, skin has no gender. It doesn't know if it is male or female and, judging from the male skins I see around, they could thrive on a little more care and attention.

Green mulch masks are very easy to make using fresh herbs. Simply put two handfuls of the appropriate herb in a liquidizer with two tablespoons of water (preferably mineral water). Blend on high speed for a few seconds. Switch off. Push any unblended herbs down from the side of the goblet with a spatula. Blend again, adding a little more water if necessary. If you've overdone the water, strain out any excess through a nylon sieve and add it to your rinse water after the mask.

Dried herbs can be used in the same way but must first be macerated in just enough boiling water to cover for several hours (this softens them). Blend the whole mixture in a liquidizer. Strain off excess liquid as above. Apply these mulches to the face in a thick layer and keep very still for twenty minutes. If you find the mask too slippery and green sludge is dripping down your neck, contain the herbs in thin pieces of gauze and apply as a poultice (see p. 34). This controls them without blocking their action on the skin.

Ideally, herbal masks should be used on a face which has been deeply cleansed and they should always be applied over a slightly damp skin. Leave them on for ten to thirty minutes and take advantage of this gap to lie down and get your feet higher than your face so that your blood flows into your face and tones up the skin. The mask can then be palmed off with damp hands unless it is a stiff one for which you need lots of warm water and a flannel. You could also use the water left over from a facial steam, which should first be strained and then allowed to cool. Be careful not to leave any bits in your hairline, eyebrows or round your ears.

Only make up two tablespoons of dried mask or three handfuls of fresh mask at a time – extra bits saved in the fridge tend to end up as unused anonymous mouldy lumps. Concocting a herbal face mask can be very creative. First decide what you want in it, bearing in mind your skin type. For example, runny honey is hydroscopic and therefore very good for skins in need of moisture as well as healing. All citrus fruits are toning, astringent and antiseptic. Grapes, apples and pears are moisturizing and nourishing; strawberries, blackcurrants, raspberries, cucumber, pumpkins and marrow soften the skin and reduce oiliness, apricots, peaches, tangerines and melons refine coarse skin; cereals and nuts whiten, soften and smooth the skin as well as contributing their own natural oils; kaolin and fuller's earth absorb oil and tighten the skin; egg white, buttermilk and yoghurt contain lactic acid which dries and tightens the skin; simple tinctures of benzoin and myrrh help to close pores; and brewer's yeast stimulates the circulation, helps healing and brings a rosy glow to your cheeks. (Madame de Pompadour brought a rosy glow to hers by covering them with beef steaks, and raw meat was also quite popular as a mask between the sixteenth and eighteenth centuries. The thought of dead flesh on my own outer layer of dead flesh nauseates me, so you won't find any meat masks in this book.)

Carrot and Marshmallow Mask (for dry, sensitive skins)

Take one large raw carrot (preferably not covered with pesticide) and grate it finely. Pound up two marshmallow leaves and stir this into the mixture with a beaten egg yolk and just enough double cream to make it into a firm slush. The carrots are full of vitamin A, which will help to clear away blemishes and the marshmallow will soothe any redness out of the skin.

Tone with diluted houseleek juice, which is superb for sore chapped skin and spots. This can be easily made by liquidizing twelve houseleek leaves with 200 ml (7 fl oz) of water. The mixture should then be strained through coffee filter paper. As you will never be able to get dried houseleek and it is not often found growing wild, your best plan is to buy a plant from a herb farm and grow it yourself. The leaves of the plant are thick, juicy, pale green and edged with purple, and the plants themselves grow in compact rose-like tufts directly from the roots. Houseleeks are best planted in the cracks of an old wall rather than in a garden bed, which they object to. (Centuries ago they were, in fact, planted on roofs.) Once established they thrive and spread very quickly by sending out offsets. I have grown houseleeks indoors in a large flat china basin containing only a few inches of soil. The beauty of houseleeks is that they seem to thrive on poor soil and neglect and once established seem practically indestructible. Houseleek was one of the most cherished cosmetic herbs of Ninon de l'Enclos who up to her death at the age of ninety-one was still called 'the woman who never grew old' and who even in her eighties was still managing to attract ardent young lovers. She almost committed incest with her grandson at the age of seventy and by all accounts led an exciting and scandalous life as a courtesan, gourmet and friend to Molière, Voltaire and Scarron.

Green Gunk Mask (for dry, sensitive skins)

Remove the skin from a tablespoon of almonds by immersing them in boiling water for a few minutes. Drain them and then squeeze the fattest end of the nut with two fingers. The nut will pop obligingly out of its skin. Pulverize the almonds in a liquidizer, then add a tablespoon of fresh parsley, two comfrey leaves, a thin slice of melon and a tablespoon of any herbal syrup. Blend again. The result will look green, sloppy and ominous (hence the name of the mask). If the mask is too sloppy strain off some of the juice. Massage this well into the skin. The abrasive action of the almonds will act as a gentle exfoliant. Tone with marshmallow milk or any strained-out excess juice from the mask.

Sir Hugh Platt recommended milk for delicate sensitive skin:

'Wash the face and body of a sucking childe with breast milke, or cow milke, or mixed with water, every night: and the child's skin will wax fair and cleare, and resist Sun burning'.

Delightes for Ladies, 1594

Tomato Mask (for oily skins)

Immerse two tomatoes briefly in hot water until their skins crack. Peel off the skin, quarter the tomatoes, scoop out the seeds and put all the flesh in a mortar. Add a tablespoon of peppermint leaves and half a tablespoon of dried yeast grains. Do not use fresh yeast in this instance; it draws the skin too severely. Pound this all together to a paste. Stir in a teaspoon of lemon juice and spread thickly on the face and neck, keeping well clear of the eye area. Tone the pores with diluted cider vinegar, 1:6.

Fennel Seed Mask (for oily skins)

Pound a tablespoon of fennel seeds to a powder. Add a tablespoon of fuller's earth and moisturize with a double-strength infusion of yarrow – enough to bind the whole into a slushy paste. Cleanse the face and tone the pores with the remaining yarrow water.

Lupin Mask (for oily skins)

Pound two tablespoons of lupin seeds to a powder or pulverize them in your liquidizer. Add enough fresh lemon juice to form a thick paste. This is a variation on John Parkinson's recommendation for removing smallpox scars and making the ladies' looks, as he put it, 'more amiable': 'use the meale of lupins mingled with the gall of a goate and some juyce of lemons to make it into the forme of a soft ointment'. As gall of goats is hard to come by I have missed it out. This mask makes a superb exfoliant as the seeds still remain slightly gritty so massage it well into the face paying special attention to greasy noses, chins and foreheads. Tone with diluted witchhazel, 1:6.

Masks for Combination Skins

Tedious as it may sound, and indeed as it is, you can use any of the above masks separately on the appropriate areas. Alternatively, try pulverizing a handful of hazelnuts which have first been roasted and then skinned with five hulled strawberries and enough plain yoghurt to form a thick paste. This has just the right balance of soothing astringency and nourishment for a combination skin and any of this mixture not used on the skin is absolutely delicious to eat afterwards!

Masks for Normal Skins

Spearmint Mask. Pound two handfuls of spearmint leaves to a paste and add a quarter of a teaspoon of any of the vitamin E-rich oils and enough of any herbal syrup to make the whole mixture spreadable. Tone with rose water.

Alternatively, spread a thin layer of home-made mayonnaise on the face (preferably one made with cider vinegar and olive oil). Rub this well into the skin and tone with very diluted Carmelite water, 1:12 (see p. 202).

Masks for Old-looking Sallow Skins in Need of a Pick-me-up

Cherry Mask. Not such a strange idea, as cherries are positively bursting with vitamins. Stone them, crush them and spread them on your face. Tone with cowslip water.

Honey Herbal Mask. Pound a tablespoon of fresh lady's mantle and a tablespoon of fresh comfrey leaves to a juicy mulch and add enough honey and wheatgerm to combine the whole. Tone with houseleek water.

A stiffly beaten egg white will tighten up saggy skin.

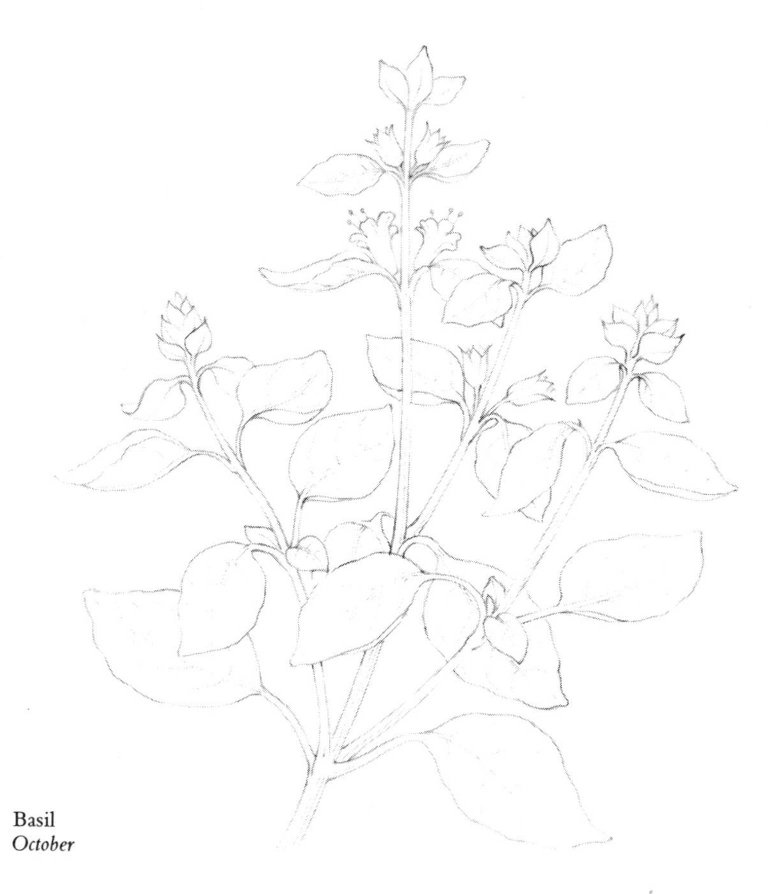

Basil
October

The milky juice from a birch tree rubbed into the skin will give it a nice glow. That is if you can get it. Called 'birch blood' by country people, it is tapped by boring a small hole in the trunk of a birch in springtime and inserting a straw into the hole. The rising sap comes up through the straw and is fed into a bucket covered with a protective cloth to stop insects dropping in. It is possible to draw as much as sixteen gallons of sap from a very large tree but the tapping has to stop after three days so as not to exhaust the tree. The hole is then stopped with a cork or a wooden plug. Tone the face with blackberry leaf water and drink lots of blackberry leaf tea. This should set you up nicely for the spring.

Scrubs

Scrubs are a very good way of exfoliating the skin and unclogging the pores. They will bring a glow to your cheeks but they should not be used by people with thread veins or open lesions on the skin.

Rose and Oatmeal Scrub (for dry and combination skins)

Mix flaky oatmeal, the bigger the flakes the better, with enough of a milk infusion of rose petals to moisten. Spread this over your face and rub the skin firmly with the flat of your fingers in small circular motions. Pay special attention to the forehead, nose and chin. Avoid the eye area. Sluice off with lots of tepid water. You may find it easier to incorporate the oatmeal and milk in a muslin bag. This should then be firmly tied up into a ball shape and used as a pad to rub the skin.

Basil Scrub (for oily and old-looking skins)

Shake most of the salt out of a handful of salted basil (for directions on how to salt herbs, see p. 21). Crush the basil in a mortar with a gentle hand. The idea is not to crush the salt too finely as the coarse crystals of salt act as a better exfoliant for this skin type. Add half a handful of flaky oatmeal and enough witchhazel to form a paste. Spread this on your face and rub the skin in a rotating movement with the flat of your fingers. Skirt around the eye area. Sluice off with lots of tepid water.

Sugar and Soapwort Scrub (for spotty, sallow skins)

Scrub a small potato. Grate it coarsely and add enough brown muscovado sugar to form a paste. Add one tablespoon of chopped soapwort. Mix and spread over the face. Rub the skin with the flats of the fingers paying special attention to the spotty areas.

It is quite a good idea to keep a small pot of these scrubs minus their liquid ingredients (and in the case of the recipe for spotty and sallow skin, minus its potato) by the wash basin, so you can use them instead of soap occasionally. For a noticeable improvement in the texture of the skin, they should be used for five days at a stretch.

Toning

Toners are particularly useful for stimulating the circulation (getting the blood up to the surface of the skin will help to nourish it), for reducing excessive oiliness and for closing the pores. Perhaps I should explain here that pores do not really open and close like doors. The words 'open' and 'close' are really a simplistic way of describing a very complex physiological action. What happens when you apply an astringent is that an edema is formed round the pore, the skin is mildly irritated causing it to puff up a bit and this makes the pore look smaller. As the effect soon dissipates it takes much patience and constant effort to get pores to look smaller all the time. Skin that looks like orange peel will only ever be temporarily redeemed.

Any herbal vinegar using a herb suitable for your skin type makes a good toner. When using a herbal vinegar always dilute 1:6 with mineral water and always use cider vinegar for your herbal vinegars if you can. Herbal wine macerations diluted again with mineral water, 6:1 are suitable toners for very delicate or old-looking skins. Herbal milks make soothing nourishing toners for very dry skin (for instructions on how to make herbal macerations, see pp. 28–31). For herbal vinegars to cure headaches, migraines and in food, see Chapter 8.

Flower waters can also be used for toning and can be used neat. They are best bought. Lavender water, rose water, orange flower water and witchhazel are readily available from good chemists. Elderflower water seems to be harder to find, so do make your own but remember it is highly perishable and should be kept in the fridge.

Elderflower Water

Gather a large handful of fresh elderflowers, bruise them gently with a pestle and mortar and pour over half a litre (1 pint) of boiling water. Transfer this mixture into a lidded jug or bowl and cover tightly. Leave to steep overnight. Strain through coffee filter paper and refrigerate. This method can be used to make any flower water. Elderflowers used to be particularly popular in the nineteenth century for refining the skin, removing freckles and keeping it blemish-free.

A blend of rose water and witchhazel with a touch of glycerine was probably used by your grandmother and her mother before her as a skin toner. Orange flower water was valued by Marie Antoinette, who used it to refine and lighten her rather sallow dark skin. It is gentler than witchhazel and suitable for delicate skins.

Simple herbal teas can be refrigerated and used as toners, if you choose a herb or blend of herbs suitable for your skin type. Make these in small quantities (see pp. 26–7) as they will not usually keep longer than three days. A teaspoon of simple tincture of benzoin or tincture of myrrh can be added to half a litre (1 pint) of herbal water intended for oily skins. This will add to its astringency and help to preserve it. A teaspoon of honey or glycerine can be dissolved in half a litre (1 pint) of warm flower water or in a herbal maceration of vinegar, water or milk to help dry delicate or chapped sore skins.

You may want to be really ambitious and construct a simple still for longer lasting herbal and flower waters.

Fill a large enamel-lined teapot or stove-kettle three quarters full of your selected herb or flower. Barely cover with water and put the lid on. Attach a rubber or, better still, a heavy plastic tube to the spout and bend the central section so that it rests in a shallow bowl of icy cold water (rubber tends to taint the herbal water slightly with its smell). Train the end of the tube over the lip of a bowl, which should be about 30 cm (12 in.) away from the teapot and at a slightly lower level than the ice water bath. Bring the contents of the teapot gently to the boil and turn down the heat so that the water is barely simmering. Continue to simmer very slowly for three quarters of an hour. As the water bubbles away, the steam rising out of the spout goes down the tube and condenses in the section that rests in the icy water. It then flows off into the collecting bowl and there is your distilled herbal water. Any such water can be further preserved by adding a few drops of simple tincture of benzoin to it.

Cucumber and Quince Lotion (for oily skins)

Bruise a large handful of quince blossom slightly, then put it in an enamel pot, cover with cold water and put the lid on. Bring to the boil and simmer for half an hour. Liquidize half a cucumber, skin and all, and add this to the pot. Simmer for a further five minutes. Strain through coffee filter paper and refrigerate. Quince blossom is now a much neglected ingredient in beauty products. A pity, really, because it is excellent for refining the pores and whitening the skin.

Strawberry Wash (for combination skins)

'Take a quart of wild strawberries, wild tansy, three pints of new Milke. Still all these together and wash your face therein.'

The Good Housewife's Handmaid, 1585

Make this up in proportionately smaller quantities. First crush the strawberries and tansy leaves with a pestle and mortar, using 60 g (2 oz) strawberries and the same weight of tansy leaves. Mix into half a litre (1 pint) of milk and leave them to macerate for an hour. Strain out the debris through a coffee filter paper. The residue can be stored in the refrigerator and will last for four to five days.

Toner (for dry, sensitive skins)

Jesemain Water
'Take two handfuls of Jeseme [Jasmine] flowers and put them into a flagon or earthen pot, put to them about a quart of fair water and a quarter of a pound of Sugar, let this stand and steep for about half an hour, then take your water and flowers and pour them out of one vessel into another till such time as the water hath taken the scent and taste of the flowers, then set it in a cool place a cooling and you will find it a most excellent scented water.'

Giles Rose (one of Charles II's master cooks), *A Perfect School of Instructions for the Officers of the Month*, 1682

You can follow the same method with rose petals, cowslips, orange, cherry or apple blossom but the fragrance cannot be compared to the ethereal smell of jasmine flowers. Diluted Carmelite water is good for normal skins, p. 202.

Toner (for old-looking sallow skins)

A Sweet Water
'Take Damask Roses at discretion, Basil, Sweet Marjoram, Lavender, Walnut Leafs, of each two handfuls, Rosemary one handful, a little Balm, Cloves, Cinnamon, one ounce, Bay leaf, Rosemary tops, Limon and Orange Pills of each a few; pour upon these as much White Wine as will conveniently wet them, and let them infuse for ten or twelve days; then distil it off.'

Sir Kenelem Digby, *Receipts in Physick and Chirurgery*, 1668

I use about two tablespoons in all of finely scraped orange and lemon peel, quills of cinnamon and whole cloves and stick to the same quantity of flowers and herbs as Digby advises. I use my home-made still to distill the mixture and the result is a delightful, fragrant, slightly spicy toner for dingy-looking skins. This is also an excellent aftershave. It keeps for nearly a year and does not need refrigerating.

William Coles advises:
'If Maids will take wilde Tansy and lay it to soak in Buttermilke for the space of nine dayes, and wash their faces therewith, it will make them look very faire'.

The Art of Simpling, 1656

Tansies are especially good for eradicating pimples and the buttermilk will refine greasy pores.

A Water to Cause an Excellent Colour and Complexion
'Drink six spoonfuls of the juice of Hyssop in warm Ale in a Morning and fasting.'

The Receipt Book of John Nott (cook to the Duke of Bolton), 1723

I should think the warm ale might have something to do with bringing a glow to your cheeks!

Moisturizing

Now on to the all-important subject of moisturizing. Reminding you yet again of the fact that the outer layers of the skin are dead may sound unnecessary but, if you grasp this, you will understand the vital necessity for moisturizing the skin. It is only the new and living cells produced deep within the epidermis that are plump and full of water. On their journey to the skin's surface they lose all their moisture and emerge flattened and desiccated. Water is the only thing that will plump them up again, making the skin feel soft and smooth, and this water must be applied externally. If it is not the skin will appear dull and lifeless. This is why I always suggest that before applying a moisturizer a thin layer of plain, herbal or flower water is patted on to the skin and left to sink in for a few seconds, only after which the moisturizer is spread, holding the precious moisture in the skin like a piece of cling film.

Lady's Mantle Moisturizer (for dry, sensitive skins)

30 g (1 oz) anhydrous lanolin

100 ml ($3\frac{1}{3}$ fl oz) almond oil

20 ml ($\frac{2}{3}$ fl oz or 4 tsp) wheatgerm oil

30 g (1 oz) lady's mantle infused in 2 cups boiling water for half an hour. Cooled, strained and 30 ml (1 fl oz) of the infusion measured out

3–6 drops essential oil of violets using the fragrant variety *Viola odorata* not dog violets which are scentless

Follow the Basic Cream Directions on p. 57.

Lettuce Moisturizer (for normal skins)

60 g (2 oz) of any lettuce variety except Chinese

30 g (1 oz) anhydrous lanolin

70 ml ($2\frac{1}{3}$ fl oz) avocado oil

10 ml ($\frac{1}{3}$ fl oz or 2 tsp) wheatgerm oil

3–6 drops essential oil of roses

Boil the lettuce in 2 cups of water for 15 minutes, and leave it to cool. Strain it, mashing the lettuce well down with a wooden spoon and measure out 30 ml (1 fl oz) of the liquid. Proceed with the Basic Cream Directions.

Chamomile Moisturizer (for combination skins)

15 g ($\frac{1}{2}$ oz) anhydrous lanolin

15 g (½ oz) beeswax

100 ml (3⅓ fl oz) safflower oil

20 ml (⅔ fl oz or 4 tsp) wheatgerm oil

30 g (1 oz) rose petals infused in 2 cups boiling water for 20 minutes. Cooled, strained and 30 ml (1 fl oz) of the infusion measured out or 30 ml (1 fl oz) rose water

3–6 drops essential oil of chamomile

3 drops simple tincture of benzoin

Follow the Basic Cream Directions on p. 57.

Liquorice Moisturizer (for old-looking skins)

30 g (1 oz) cocoa butter

30 g (1 oz) anhydrous lanolin

100 ml (3⅓ fl oz) avocado oil

20 ml (⅔ fl oz or 4 tsp) wheatgerm oil

30 g (1 oz) chopped liquorice root simmered in 1½ cups water for 45 minutes. Cooled, strained and 30 ml (1 fl oz) of the decoction measured out

3–6 drops lavender oil

Follow the Basic Cream Directions on p. 57.

Blackberry Lotion (for oily skins)

Never make the mistake of thinking an oily skin does not need a moisturizer. Its problem is too much oil, not too much water, and it needs just as much protection as any other skin.

30 g (1 oz) beeswax

90 ml (3 fl oz) peach kernel oil

10 ml (⅓ fl oz or 2 tsp) wheatgerm oil

15 g (½ oz) blackberry leaves infused in 1 cup water for 30 minutes. Cooled, strained and 15 ml (½ fl oz or 1 tbsp) measured out

15 ml (½ fl oz or 1 tbsp) witchhazel

3 drops essential oil of marigold

2 drops tincture of myrrh

Follow the Basic Lotion Directions on p. 58.

An oily skin need only be moisturized with tiny blobs of this lotion. Pay special attention to areas around the eyes and mouth, and to the throat. Let it sink into the skin for ten minutes, then blot off any excess, especially on the nose and forehead, with a tissue before applying foundation or powder.

Strawberry Milk Moisturizer (for chapped skins)

I made this for someone who had returned from a climbing expedition with very sore chapped skin. It is very soothing and healing and because it is so light does not drag across the sore skin and make it worse:

'Take a small Handful of Strawberry Leaves, as much Cinquefoil, the same quantity of Tansey or of Mallows, and four Handfuls of Plantane Leaves, pick them clean, put them into an Alembick and also two quarts of Milk from the Cow, when it has dropped a quart, draw off no more. Wet a Linen Cloth in this distilled Water and wash the Face with it, at Night in Bed, and several times during the day if you please. The best time to make this Water in is May. It may be kept in a glass Bottle the whole year.'

Charles Carter (cook to the Duke of Argyll) *The Compleat City and Country Cook*, 1732

I do not know about its keeping properties. My climber used it up too quickly for me to find out, but even after distillation in an 'Alembick' I should think a year was a bit on the optimistic side! I used my home-made still and kept the mixture in the refrigerator for a week until it was finished.

Mayonnaise Skin Food

1 large raw egg yolk

4 tbsp cider vinegar

½ cup corn oil

3 tbsp wheatgerm oil

4 tsp double-strength decoction of marshmallow root

1 tsp clear honey

This is most easily made in a liquidizer. First, blend the egg yolk and half the vinegar. Now slowly, slowly trickle in half the corn oil and when it is well amalgamated add the rest of the vinegar, the marshmallow decoction and the honey. Again slowly, add the remaining oil, including the wheatgerm oil. Keep the mixture in your refrigerator. It makes a magnificent skin food, which should be used sparingly at night. Blot off any excess oil with tissues. It also makes an excellent lotion which can be used to soften and lubricate skin before taking a bath. The warm water will wash off any excessive oil and the skin is left feeling smooth and silky. Surprisingly, and happily, the mayonnaise does not smell at all unpleasant and it is not like sleeping with a salad, as my husband observed with relief when he first found me trying it.

Chapter 3
Groom and Bloom

Eyes

If your eyes are the windows of the soul it would be just as well to present your soul at its best – shining, happy and unclouded by redness, puffiness and shadows. Enough sleep to suit your own needs is the first most important prerequisite for sparkling eyes. Some people can manage on five hours nightly, other people need ten. I have even met someone who practised yoga and meditation at intervals throughout the day and night and claimed he could manage without any sleep at all. Find your own needs and stick to them as far as you can. If you have to cut down on one night's ration catch up the next night. Insomniacs will be helped by the suggestions in Chapter 8.

The incontinent use of drugs, alcohol and tobacco will inevitably take their toll on the eyes as will a poor diet. Vitamin A, which is fat-soluble and cannot be stored by the body, is the eye vitamin, so make sure you have a daily dose: dandelion leaves are an excellent herbal source of vitamin A. Silicon is the mineral which contributes to healthy eyesight – people who feel their eyesight is deteriorating often suffer from a shortage of silicon. Herbal sources of silicon are horsetail, comfrey, dandelion, nettles, hound's tongue and lungwort.

Herbal Eye Washes to Refresh Tired Eyes

Herbal eye washes should always be made up and used as soon as they have cooled. Any residue should be fed to houseplants or the compost heap, not stored. There is no point in introducing infections to perfectly healthy if somewhat tired eyes. Compresses soaked in herbal eye washes should always be kept scrupulously clean. Do not re-use them. Throw them away. If you find you are constantly having to use eye washes consult a doctor. A prolonged need for them may mean you have much more serious eye problems than a simple need to refresh tired, sore eyes. Try to avoid the temptation of rubbing your eyes with your hands. Eyes are highly susceptible to infection. If you simply must rub use a clean tissue and be gentle.

Use a decoction, not an infusion, of any of the herbs below. The prolonged boiling of a decoction will ensure that nearly all bacteria are killed. Make sure that you strain all decoctions intended for the eyes at least three times through coffee filter paper. This precaution ensures there are no bits left to float around in your eyes.

angelica seeds
borage
eyebright
cornflower blossom
cotton lavender
fennel seeds
greater celandine
hyssop
lady smocks
poppy seed capsules (use 3 capsules to a quarter of a litre of water, simmering for 5 minutes)
rose water
wild clary sage seed

Wood betony can also be taken internally as a tea to relieve sore eyes. Be very careful you do not confuse angelica with hemlock. The two plants are part of the same family but hemlock contains a poisonous principle, conine.

The Arabs have used the juice crushed from cotton lavender for centuries as eye drops to soothe and protect the eyes from searing, gritty desert wind. They also mix the juice with chilled milk and apply it on eye pads to reduce puffiness.

Eyebright is probably one of the best known herbs for the eyes. The French call it *casse-lunette* because they feel so many people are able to throw away their spectacles after its prolonged use. Culpeper observed 'if the herb was but as much used as it is neglected, it would spoil the spectacle-makers' trade'. The Germans call it *Augentröst* (consolation to the eyes) and the Italians *luminella* (light for the eyes). I use angelica, fennel and witchhazel in my own eye balm as I find them the ideal combination for tired, irritated puffy eyes. Make sure that if you wear contact lenses you remove them before using an eye wash or a compress.

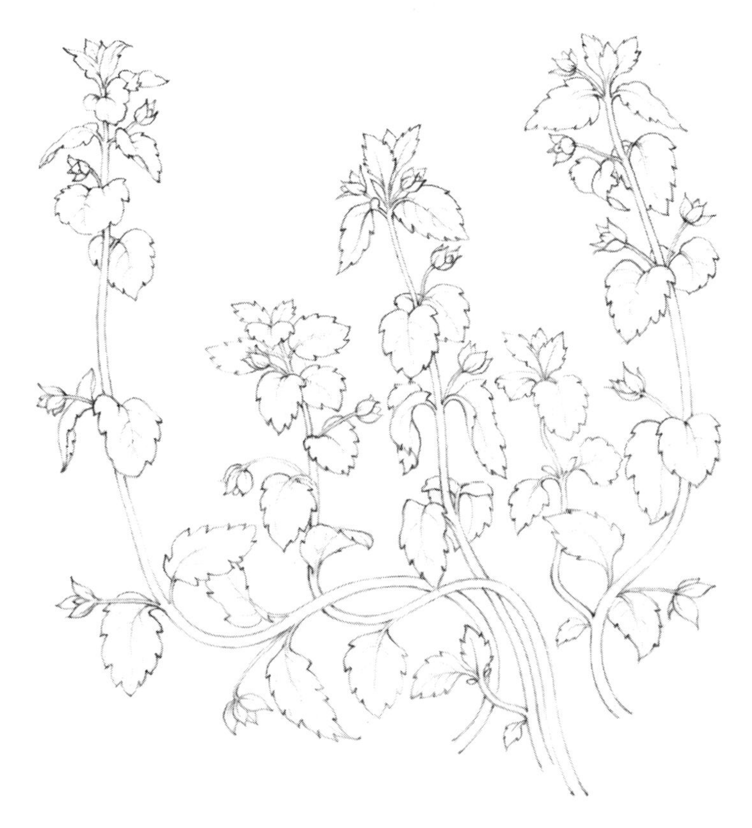

Eyebright
October

Herbal Eye Pads to Refresh Tired Eyes and Reduce Puffiness

Thinly sliced chilled cucumber.

Thinly sliced potato, scrubbed and first peeled (to get very thin slices use a mandoline).

Grated raw apple, spread on a piece of gauze and placed gauze side down on the eyelids.

Barely wet lukewarm tea bags.

Fennel seed compress.

Witchhazel compress. To protect your eyes from the stinging of the witchhazel first rub the eyelid and the surrounding area with a thin film of wheatgerm oil and then apply the pad.

A double-strength decoction of eyebright, filtered three times and poured into an ice cube tray. Freeze. Store the frozen cubes in a plastic bag and use one to rub over the eyes when you feel in need of it. Holding the cube in a piece of thick lint will prevent frozen fingertips.

Obviously, all these solutions should not be used together. Try one at a time until you find the recipe which is most beneficial for you.

Herbal Methods to Reduce Inflammation and Help Watering Eyes

Remember to use a decoction, not an infusion, of any of the following herbs:

Chervil water.

Cornflower blossom.

Muslin bags filled with chickweed, tied, plunged into boiling water for two minutes, cooled and then placed on the eyelids.

Poppy flower compress.

Compress of scarlet pimpernel smeared with a little clear honey.

Gerard said that a decoction of meadowsweet 'dropped into the eyes takes away the burning and itching there of'.

One part of a decoction of greater celandine, using the leaves, the stem and the flowers too if possible mixed with three parts of a decoction of rose petals helps to clear the whites of the eyes.

Lime blossom taken internally and used as an eye wash externally is good for muscular weakness of the eyes. Make sure the flowers used are freshly picked, or if you use dried flowers that they are not more than a month old. Stale flowers can produce symptoms of narcotic intoxication.

Raspberry leaves, walnut leaves, wormwood, marshmallow roots and melilot are also good herbal remedies for inflamed eyes.

Stye Removers

Macerate 60 g (2 oz) of fresh or 15 g ($\frac{1}{2}$ oz) dried walnut leaves in a litre (1$\frac{3}{4}$ pints) of cold water for four hours. Bring slowly to the boil and simmer for two minutes. Leave to infuse for a further fifteen minutes. Strain several times through coffee filter paper. Bottle in a sterilized jar and dab this lotion on the stye repeatedly with cotton wool. Twice daily use the lotion as a compress.

Horsetail is not only excellent for styes but cures the swelling of the tear ducts and general tenderness of the eyes. Follow exactly the same method as for walnut leaves, using the same quantity of herb but boiling for half an hour instead of two minutes.

Pound up a teaspoon of nasturtium seeds to a gritty paste. Spread these on a piece of freshly boiled gauze. Allow the poultice to cool to lukewarm, then gently place over the stye, gauze side innermost, rather like an open sandwich. Leave until cool. Remove. Repeat as often as possible during the course of the day and at least twice daily.

All of the above recipes for removing styes can be made from the dried equivalents and, as styes are no respecters of seasons, it would be as well to keep some of these dried herbs aside in case of emergency (see p. 24 for quantities of dried herbs).

To Remove Foreign Bodies from the Eyes

Coles, in *The Art of Simpling*, recommends:

the seeds of Clary, but especially of the wild sort, which is called Oculus Christi, one of which being put into each Eye cleareth them, and purgeth them exceedingly from waterish humours, rednesse and inflammation and other divers maladies, if not all that happen unto the Eyes, and taketh away the paine and smarting of.

You would be well advised not to put the seed directly into the eye. Make a decoction instead and bathe the eyes in this using an eye bath. The two next treatments I have not tried but for centuries they have been judged successful by the peoples who use them.

The North American Indians make up a decoction of the root and the leaves of the pitcher plant which they believe helps to relieve the sensation of black spots floating in front of the eyes.

The Arabs use sap extracted from the vine, called a 'tear' or 'lachryma', in the belief that it helps to remove specks on the cornea and strengthens weak eyes.

To Sharpen Eyesight

A Distilled Water for strengthening the Sight

'Take Rosemary flowers, Sage, Betony, Rue and Succory, of each 1 handful. Infuse these in 2 quarts of good Sack, distill them in a Copper Alembick. The Dose is a moderate spoonful.'

The Honourable R. Boyle, F.R.S., *Medicinal Experiments, or, A Collection of Choice and Safe Remedies*, 1718

The high alcoholic content of this recipe might at least bring a sparkle to the eyes if you took more than a mere moderate spoonful and certainly rue is a herb that was used centuries ago by engravers, carvers and painters, who depended on the sharpness of their eyesight to make a living.

Rue Lotion to Sharpen the Eyesight

1 tbsp rue flowers

½ tsp white wine

60 ml (2 fl oz) mineral water

Put all ingredients in a glass bowl placed over a pot of boiling water. Cover with a plate. Allow the lotion to heat gently for two hours, remembering to top up the boiling water in the pot from time to time. Allow to cool still covered. Strain through coffee filter paper. Immediately store in a sterilized container. Use this lotion as an eye bath to bathe the eyes twice daily. This mixture should last about two days. It will have to be used for several weeks before any improvement is noticed.

Dark Circles and Puffiness

Sad to say, bags and dark circles under the eyes are often hereditary. Mind you, they are not helped by lack of sleep or excessive nervous strain. Puffiness under the eyes tends to accelerate with age because the skin in this area is thinner and more delicate than anywhere else on the body.

As with all skin care problems prevention is better than cure.

Raise your bed up at the head end by 10 cm (4 in.) and sleep with a neck roll instead of a pillow.

To encourage any excess fluid which may have accumulated in this area to drain away drink lots of depurative teas (see p. 177).

Use daily a poultice of grated potato. Try a poppy, rosehip or chamomile compress (p. 32). Do not take chamomile more than twice weekly as it can result in irritation if used over too long a period at a time. Alternate with the other herbs.

Apply a poultice of one fresh fig, divided in half, slightly mashed and laid between four pieces of gauze (two for each eye). Leave on for twenty minutes.

Conjunctivitis

This can be extremely painful and should be treated with tepid compresses of any one of the following herbs – cornflower blossom, plantain, elder leaves and, above all, eyebright – applied up to five times daily. Ice cold compresses will shock sore eyes too much. While the condition lasts drink two tablespoons of the following tea twice daily:

Rue Tea

½ level tsp dried rue

60 ml (2 fl oz) water

Pour the freshly boiled water over the herb. Cover and allow to steep for two hours. Strain and drink as directed. If it tastes too bitter to be palatable sweeten with honey while still warm. Rue is a very potent herb so follow directions on dosage exactly. Do not take immediately after a meal as it also acts as an emetic.

From cream suitable for below the eyes, see p. 166. Never rub any essential herbal oil directly on to the eyelids or under the eyes. If you want to treat yourself to a simple eye oil add one drop of essential oil of fennel, angelica or lavender to 60 ml (2 fl oz) of wheatgerm oil. Shake the bottle before each use and apply nightly, spreading a tiny drop lightly over the area beneath the eye. Blot off any excess with tissues after you have allowed it to sink into the skin for ten minutes.

Eyebrow Conditioner

Using a child's toothbrush lightly brush on a double-strength decoction of sage. After several applications the eyebrows will turn darker. Unruly eyebrows can be tamed by using one tablespoon of almond oil mixed with three drops of essential oil of sage or southernwood. Dip the toothbrush in this mixture and comb the hairs in the direction you want them to lie.

Eyelash Conditioner

This treatment not only conditions the eyelashes but in some instances helps them grow longer and thicker. Patience and nightly application will show results. Brush your lashes nightly with a scrupulously clean mascara brush dipped in almond or castor oil. Be very careful not to drip the oil into the eyes. If you do so it will make your eyes smart and your vision blurry for a while. This is not serious; it is just inconvenient.

Exercises for the Eyes

Rub your palms together hard so that the friction generates some heat. Cup your palms over your eyes, fingers pointing upwards to the hairline. Let your eyes bask in the warmth and darkness of the palms. Stay like this until the heat has disappeared. Now trail your fingers gently across your eyes from the inner corners to the temples. Do this several times.

Pretend you have a very large clock right in front of your eyes, with the numbers of the hours painted right at the edge. Starting at twelve o'clock very slowly move your eyes from one hour to the next in a clockwise direction, pausing for a second at each number. Do not move your head. Once you reach twelve o'clock pause, then begin the exercise again moving your eyes in an anti-clockwise direction.

Roll your head and neck in the largest circle you can manage without moving your shoulders. Don't strain and don't exaggerate your movements. At first the neck muscles may feel so tight that your head is confined to sketching a very small circle. Practice will loosen the muscles and make the exercise easier. This not only improves vision by increasing the circulation to the optic nerves, but it relaxes the entire upper body and eases shoulder strain.

All these exercises work extremely well to relax the strain engendered by prolonged periods of close reading or writing.

Crow's feet

Beat one egg white with one teaspoon of honey until frothy. Pat on the crow's feet. Let it dry and sponge off gently with a decoction of fennel. Pat on a tiny amount of wheatgerm oil.

For wrinkled eyelids apply a compress of freshly squeezed orange juice mixed half-and-half with a double-strength decoction of eyebright. Leave it on for half an hour. Do not wash it off. Pat on wheatgerm oil or apply the mayonnaise cream on p. 80.

Stir enough double cream into an egg white to make the mixture spreadable. Leave on the crow's feet at least an hour or all night if possible. Wash off with tepid chamomile tea.

Mouth and Teeth

Oral Hygiene

To most people halitosis is a fate worse than leprosy. Food particles in the teeth do not cause bad breath in themselves, but once combined with oral bacteria plaque builds up. If left unchecked a very unpleasant condition called 'trench mouth' may well be the result. The food you eat can also cause bad breath: garlic, for example, is notorious for lingering for days as it is absorbed into the blood stream and exuded through the lungs. Eating a small bunch of parsley, basil, thyme or any of the mints will help to blot up the fumes before they can be released, but eat any of these herbs as soon after eating the garlic as you can.

Mouth washes help sweeten the breath, but only temporarily. Get to the root of the problem by following a diet which includes lots of chlorophyll and being meticulous about oral hygiene. Make sure you are not suffering from constipation, which can also cause bad breath. If halitosis persists, see a doctor or dentist. Of those people over thirty who still have their teeth (and one third do not) three out of four have some periodontal disease. Periodontal disease is the most widespread disease in the world. It is often relatively painless and therefore symptomless until it is well-advanced. Bleeding gums are one of the first ominous signs and unhappily most people tend to ignore them, believing it is the overzealous use of a toothbrush which is causing them. Do not be deceived. See your dentist immediately. The bacterial plaque which is mostly responsible for the bleeding can be carefully and effectively removed by your dentist.

Herbal Mouth Rinses

Verbena infusion helps not only to sweeten the breath but is believed to help resistance to tooth decay if used in conjunction with meticulous oral hygiene. It smells and tastes lovely.

Lavender and violet infusions are both excellent antiseptic herbs.

Chewing a stick of cinnamon or a clove is an instant powerful breath freshener.

Tincture of myrrh helps to strengthen and disinfect spongy gums if added to any of the herbal mouth rinses listed above. Three drops to each cup is sufficient.

Correct Tooth Brushing

Do not brush your teeth in a straight up-and-down movement, the way I was taught to do when I was a little girl. Instead, use a soft brush with rounded bristles spread with a

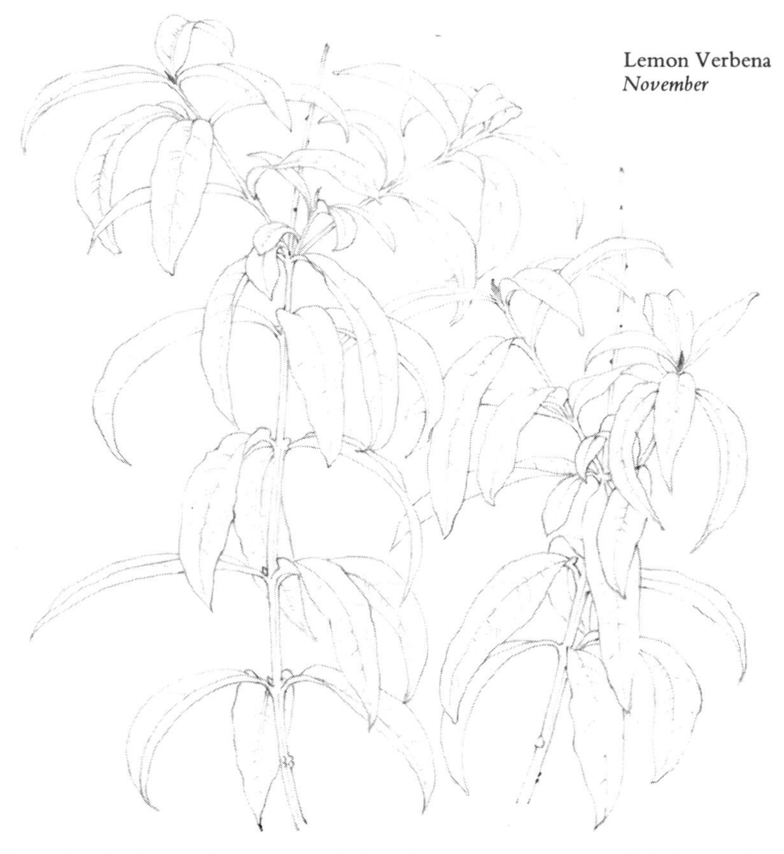

Lemon Verbena
November

little herbal toothpaste and hold it at an angle of 45° to the tooth. Scrub gently following this angle. Rinse out the mouth. Now dislodge the plaque from between the teeth with dental floss. (Plaque is the main carrier of acid-producing bacteria which attack the calcium content of the teeth and cause decay.) Repeat the brushing process using more toothpaste. Finally, massage your gums in small rotating circles with your fingertips. The use of dental floss takes a little time if done properly and is best carried out at night. Dental floss reaches the areas where the brush cannot penetrate and therefore daily flossing is essential. There is absolutely no point in using a hard toothbrush as it only wears away the enamel on teeth and encourages gum recession.

Teeth should be thoroughly brushed at least once a day. The modern school of thought as far as brushing goes tends to place the emphasis on how long rather than how often, so spend four to five minutes really concentrating on careful brushing. You should carry out a really thorough clean once a day together with the use of dental floss.

Herbal Toothpicks and Gum Massagers

These can be made with marshmallow root or liquorice root. Clean a 5 cm (2 in.) piece of root. Boil it hard in water until it just begins to soften. Drain. Allow to cool, then carefully shape the end into a rounded point with a sharp knife. Moisten the tip well with saliva before using and use once only before throwing away. The liquorice, particularly, tastes lovely and helps to sweeten the breath. Use cautiously so that the stick does not splinter and prick your gum. These are not suitable for people with tender gums or for children.

Natural Tooth Cleaners

Dentists now believe that ending a meal with cheese or peanuts is a most effective way of cleaning the teeth with natural foods. Both leave the mouth in a non-acidic condition which is less likely to help corrosion than the acid left in the mouth by munching apples, carrots or celery.

Fresh sage leaves scrubbed on teeth have been used to good effect for centuries by the Arabs. Simply pick a leaf and rub it over the teeth. Discard it as soon as it begins to get soggy and move on to a new one. Three or four leaves should be enough to polish all the teeth and make your mouth smell sweet.

For teeth that are yellow
'Take Sage and Salt, of each alike, and stampe them well together, then bake it till it be hard, and make a fine powder thereof, then therewith rub the teeth evening and morning, and it will take away all yellownesse.'

Gervase Markham, *Countrey Contentments*, 1623

Use fine sea salt and, if possible, fresh sage which in this instance works better than dried.

This is a superb toothpowder and it does help to remove nicotine stains from the teeth. Whiteness or yellowness of the teeth is inherited. Naturally, yellow teeth will never become white even with the most studious care, but, by way of compensation, the darkest yellow teeth are often the strongest and most decay-resistant.

Powdered orris root and powdered charcoal mixed in equal quantities also make an effective toothpaste. Add a few drops of clove or peppermint oil to help mask the flavour.

Never use abrasives like pumice stone or cuttlefish bone on the teeth. Their abrasive action will gradually wear away the enamel.

Teething

Babies should be enticed to chew on a boiled marshmallow root. Enticed is the right word as it is difficult to get them to oblige, but if you can manage it it does relieve the pain very quickly.

Toothache

Put a drop of essential oil of cloves into the tooth and rub another into the gum round the tooth. Repeat as often as necessary. Alternatively, macerate whole cloves in warm honey for at least half an hour. Warm the honey by heating on the stove first, then transfer it to the airing cupboard to keep it warm. Chew the cloves slowly, rolling them round the aching tooth with your tongue.

Chew a yarrow leaf using the tooth or teeth that are causing the pain.

Rub essential oil of marjoram or pennyroyal into the cavity in the aching tooth and into the surrounding gum.

As an emergency measure you can plug any cavity with a tiny sliver of fresh horseradish root or garlic (both of which are powerfully antiseptic) until you see a dentist; although my own dentist ruefully observed that it might be kinder to the dentist to use chewing gum.

For Toothake
'Take two or three Docke rootes, and as many Daisie rootes, and boyle them in water till they be soft, then take them out of the water, and boyle them well over again in oile Olive, then straine them thorow a clean cloth, and annoynt the pained tooth therewith, and keepe your mouth close, and it will not only take away the paine but also ease any megrin or griefe of the head.'

Gervase Markham, *Countrey Contentments*, 1623

Gingivitis and Periodontitis

If your gums start bleeding with only the slightest pressure get to your dentist as fast as you can. Meanwhile, use double-strength decoctions of any of the following herbs as a mouth wash:

- agrimony
- bistort
- cornflower blossom
- cowslips
- marshmallow
- rosehips

Sore Throats

Gargle with double-strength decoctions of any of the following herbs:

- blackberry leaves
- hawthorn
- hollyhock
- sage
- thyme
- vervain

I treat sore throats among my staff very successfully with

gargles of sage and honey. Sip a small glass of freshly squeezed pineapple or blackcurrant juice often throughout the day as long as the soreness persists.

Gumboils and Mouth Ulcers

Whichever one of the following remedies you choose, be prepared to persist with the treatment for at least seven to ten days, before the ulcer finally heals.

Rub the sore with the following lotion:

6 drops essential oil of coltsfoot

3 drops tincture of myrrh

½ tsp honey

Drink a decoction of equal parts of liquorice and comfrey root, swooshing it round the mouth before swallowing.

Pound up a crushed custard apple leaf and apply it to the sore as a poultice. If you wrap the pulp in a tiny strip of gauze it will help to keep it in place. When I was a little girl my ayah used to treat gumboils with this African remedy.

Add a teaspoon of salt to a quarter of a litre (half a pint) of warm water and use as a mouth wash. Any antiseptic mouth wash will reduce the risk of secondary infection but do seek the advice of a dentist as quickly as you can.

Hair and Scalp

You should treat your hair and scalp with the same sort of care and gentleness you lavish on your skin.

Hair Care

Start from the inside out by nourishing your body with the right food. Make sure you are getting enough of the B complex vitamins, as well as vitamins A and C, and iron, iodine and copper. Iodine is especially important as it is needed for proper functioning of the thyroid gland, which in turn encourages efficient scalp circulation. If the circulation is sluggish in the scalp the hair may start to weaken and fall out. Herbal sources of iodine include bladderwrack, garlic and kelp. People who are very overweight should be careful not to take too much as an excess of iodine is very toxic: 150 micrograms – a small but vital amount which is the equivalent of two teaspoons of powdered kelp – will cover your daily requirements.

Select a brush which will move through your dry hair as easily as a wide-toothed comb. Natural bristle brushes tend to be too soft to stimulate the scalp and their closely packed bristles often tug at and damage the hair. The ideal brush has well-spaced nylon bristles with rounded ends and a flexible rubber base which can be easily washed.

Use a non-metal comb without jagged teeth which will gouge and damage your scalp. Make sure the teeth are widely spaced. The only instance in which a wide-toothed aluminium comb may be of use is if your hair contains lots of static electricity.

Encourage efficient scalp circulation by massaging your scalp daily with your fingertips. Tense your fingers and, starting at the nape of your neck, work towards your forehead in small rotating circles.

Protect your hair from the sun and salt wind with hats or scarves. Chlorine encourages the loss of iodine from the body so if you are swimming in a chlorinated pool wear a bathing cap. If you must swim in the sea without a cap remember to rinse all the salt out of your hair as soon as you come out. Failing this, at least towel it dry and protect it with a scarf.

Avoid chemical rinses, tints, bleaches and perms. There are gentle herbal methods of changing your hair colouring.

Shampoo regularly with a mild herbal shampoo and always follow it with an acidified herbal rinse or conditioner. Most people use far too much shampoo. Start with a quarter of what you think you may need and work up very slowly from there. One to two teaspoons is usually ample. Rinse, rinse and rinse again after shampooing. This is just as important as the shampooing process itself. Contrary to popular belief you do not need a shampoo down the low end of the pH scale which is highly acid as it is actually possible to over-acidify your hair. The emphasis should lie on the mild qualities of the shampoo and the mildest shampoos available are the ones you can make yourself with herbs.

Never use very hot hood dryers and if you use a hand dryer hold it at least 10 cm (4 in.) away from the hair and play it lightly over the hair moving the dryer constantly. Do not treat one section to a concentrated blast. Do not use electric curlers or electrically heated tongs.

Never sleep with rollers in your hair all night. Besides stretching and breaking the hair shaft and gouging the scalp you will not get a very relaxed night's sleep.

Never use metal-toothed rollers. Use foam or plastic ones and keep them as clean as your hairbrush and comb.

Never use rubber bands or even plastic-coated ones. You can put your hair up with pretty ribbons, combs and slides instead.

It would be unrealistic to say you should never perm your hair but if you must do so don't experiment with a home perm. Go to a really good hairdresser. If a perm strips all the sheen out of your hair, condition it with a cup of black strap molasses and leave it on for at least an hour. More if you can spare the time. It is messy and may sound unlikely but it is remarkably effective. Follow this conditioner with a cider vinegar rinse.

Do not backcomb your hair.

After such an enormous list of admonitions let's consider the positive side of hair care. You can use soapwort as an entirely natural herbal shampoo for cleaning your hair or make your own gentle herbal shampoo using castile soap mixed with appropriate herbal infusions or decoctions.

To Make a Herbal Castile Shampoo

Make an infusion or decoction using 30 g (1 oz) of herbs and half a litre (1 pint) of water. Allow the brew to stand overnight, then strain out the herbs. Pour the herbal water into an enamel saucepan and add 30 g (1 oz) of grated castile soap. Heat the mixture stirring constantly until the soap has melted. Allow the shampoo to cool to lukewarm and add two drops of an appropriate herbal essential oil. Castile soap is better than a detergent-based one, which not only does a very thorough job of cleaning the hair but also strips it of all its natural oils, so don't consider taking a short cut by substituting washing up liquid.

This recipe makes enough shampoo to last for about eight sessions. If the soap content of the shampoo solidifies (and it might do under cold conditions), simply put the bottle in a warm airing cupboard until the soap melts, then shake the contents and use. Herbal shampoos should keep for at least six to eight weeks. Many will keep much longer.

Hair Herbs

Herbs for Fair Hair

chamomile

cowslips

great mullein flowers

nettles

quassia bark

quince juice expressed from the fruit by boiling in water

rhubarb root

turmeric

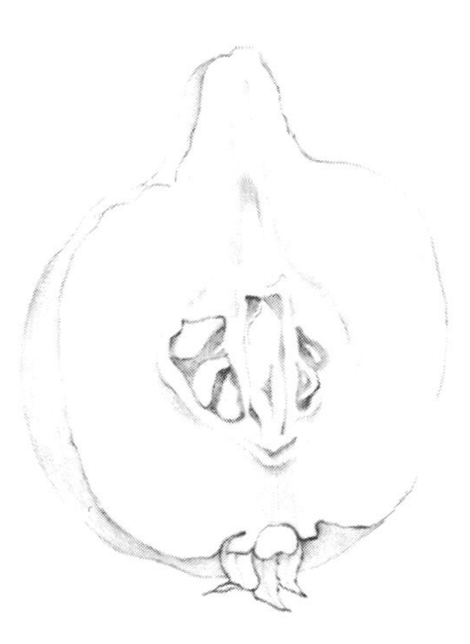

Quince
November

Herbs for Brunettes

cherry bark
cinnamon
cloves
henna
marjoram
parsley
privet

Herbs for Red Hair

ginger
henna
juniper berries
marigolds
red hibiscus
sage
witchhazel bark

Herbs for Dark Hair

elder leaves
henna
lavender
raspberry leaves
rosemary
sage
southernwood
thyme

Herbs for Conditioning Dry Hair

burdock root
comfrey
elderflowers
marshmallow
quince blossom
sage

Herbs for Conditioning Oily Hair

any of the mints
horsetail
lemon balm
lavender
marigolds
southernwood
witchhazel bark
yarrow

Suribachi with Southernwood
October

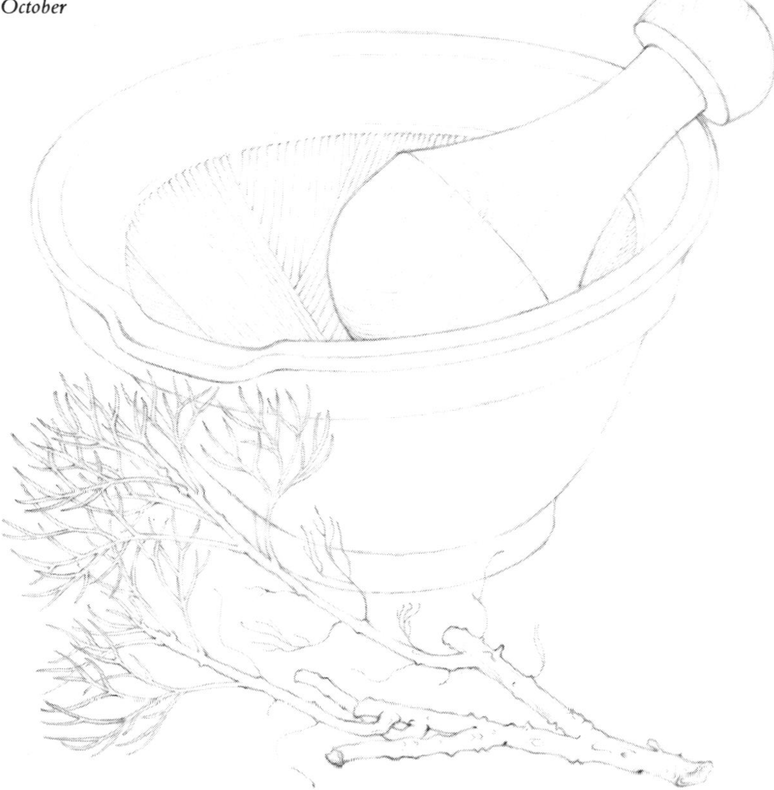

Dry Shampoos

These can never equal the thorough cleaning of a proper shampoo and water but they are useful in emergencies. The secret of a successful dry shampoo is to brush the shampoo out of the hair really thoroughly. Spend at least five minutes doing this. Even after the most thorough brushing, dry shampoos tend to leave some people with a dry scalp, so use them as infrequently as you possibly can.

Finely powdered orris root. It is possible to obtain orris root which has been sifted through a coarse mesh. Although this is the best sort to use for pot pourri-making it is not good for a dry shampoo. The finer the orris root powder the more oil-absorbing capacity it will have. Section the hair, and sprinkle on the orris root powder. Rub it lightly into the scalp with your fingertips. Now brush and brush and brush.

Finely ground almond meal or finely ground oatmeal.

Fuller's earth, preferably white. Grey fuller's earth even after conscientious brushing tends to leave the hair looking very slightly dingy.

Finely ground cornmeal.

Lavender water for very oily hair. Soak a piece of cheesecloth in the water. Force the cloth over the bristles of your brush. Keep brushing this through the hair. As soon as the cloth has accumulated a fair amount of oil and grime rinse it out thoroughly in water. Wring it out. Repeat the process until the hair is shining clean.

Rose water for dry hair. Use the same process as for lavender water.

Shampoo for Dry, Lack-lustre Hair

2 tbsp castile-based shampoo using any of the conditioning herbs for dry hair

2 egg yolks

1 tsp almond oil

Liquidize all the ingredients in a blender. Wet your hair thoroughly. Massage well into the scalp adding a little water as you go. Rinse with an appropriate herbal rinse. Condition your hair in between shampoos by spreading two drops of essential oil of chamomile or rosemary (depending on your hair colouring) on your hands. Rub the tips of the bristles of your brush over your hands so that they pick up the oil. Now brush the hair from the root to the tips in long steady strokes.

Bend over from the waist so your head hangs and your hair falls forward.

Shampoo for Oily Hair

Two tablespoons of castile-based shampoo using any of the herbs listed for oily hair. Rinse with a decoction or infusion of the same herbs mixed with a tablespoon of cider vinegar. Remember, too much shampooing only aggravates the problem of oily hair. Contrary to popular belief, brushing well does not encourage oiliness in the hair. Instead it helps distribute the oil being pumped out by the sebaceous glands evenly along the hair shaft right to the ends which are very often lacking in oil.

Help to correct oily hair by making sure you are taking in adequate daily supplies of vitamins and minerals and by drinking lots of yarrow or horsetail tea.

Herbal Hair Rinses

These are almost as important as a good herbal shampoo as they help to protect and condition the hair. Before you begin your shampooing make up an infusion or decoction of one or a mixture of herbs appropriate for your hair type using at least one scented herb to make your hair smell nice. Wait until the water has cooled to tepid, then strain out the herbs, first through a nylon sieve and then through coffee filter paper. This added precaution of using coffee filter paper is especially important as it eliminates even the finest bits of herb, which you won't want left in your hair.

After shampooing rinse your hair with lots and lots of tepid running water (this is where a shower comes in handy). Once it is entirely soap-free start pouring the herbal rinse through your hair, catching any excess in a small movable basin. Keep pouring the herbal rinse from the basin to your jug and back through your hair until your arms get tired. Now blot the hair dry with a thick towel. Gently untangle your hair with your fingers. Do not pull it. Then use your wide-toothed comb.

Herbal Rinse to Stimulate Hair Growth

1 tbsp nettles
1 tbsp jaborandi
1 tbsp marigold
1 tbsp southernwood
1 tbsp rosemary
1 tbsp watercress
1 litre (1¾ pints) water

Infuse. Add a tablespoon of cider vinegar after straining. Rinse, massaging well into the scalp.

Special Herbal Hair Treatments

Hot Oil Treatment for Dry, Damaged or Bleached Hair

1 Brush the hair vigorously, bending from the waist so that the head and the hair fall forward.

2 Choose any polyunsaturated oil such as almond, sesame, safflower, sunflower or corn oil which will penetrate the hair well. Heat up 30 ml (1 fl oz) of oil until it is lukewarm. Add six drops of rosemary, lavender or basil oil to it.

3 Wet the hair well. The water will protect the hair shaft and ensure that it is the scalp that mainly absorbs the oil.

4 Section the hair and apply oil to the scalp only, using a gauze or cotton pad. Massage it in gently with the fingertips. Pin up the rest of the hair, out of the way.

5 Now wring out a hand towel dipped in a hot infusion of any of the herbs recommended for oily hair. Wrap it around the head turban-fashion. Cover it with a big shower cap to trap the heat.

6 As soon as the scalp feels cool repeat with a fresh hot towel. If this is too tedious sit under a warm hood dryer.

7 Try and keep the treatment on for at least an hour. Two is ideal if you have the time. Do not attempt to sleep in it. You will get an awful crick in the neck.

8 Wash with a herbal shampoo for dry hair. You may need two or even three shampoos to really get the oil out of the hair.

9 Rinse with lots and lots of barely tepid water to close all the pores. Use a final rinse of any of the appropriate herbal infusions.

To save all the messing around with towels you can sit in a sauna or a Turkish bath bedaubed with the oil treatment and a shower cap to stop it dripping. This is not quite as effective as the complete treatment.

Herbal Conditioner for Oily Hair

Make no mistake about it, oily hair needs conditioning as much as dry hair, just as oily skin needs the protection of a moisturizer as much as dry skin does. An appropriate herbal rinse will usually suffice, but once a month treat yourself to the following recipe:

3 tbsp rum (white or dark, depending on your hair colouring)

3 tbsp orange flower water

1 tsp any herbal syrup, but yarrow is best

2 egg yolks (save the whites)

Liquidize all the ingredients together. Now proceed as with the previous hot oil treatment, starting at step 4 and continuing right up to step 9. Shampoo, using – strange as it may seem – the two egg whites you have saved, beaten frothy and mixed with the juice of half a lemon. Rinse with tepid water and make your final rinse an appropriate herb one. Your hair will feel glossy, manageable and super clean. If you want to set your hair use skimmed milk with a sprinkling of fine sea salt dissolved into it as your hair setting lotion.

Conditioner for Sunbleached, Wind-shredded, Salty Hair

Massage mayonnaise into the scalp and proceed as for hot oil treatment (p. 104). Rinse and shampoo with your own herbal shampoo. Make the final rinse one of equal parts of comfrey leaf and burdock root.

Problem hair is usually the result of poor nutrition, stress, prolonged illness, poor circulation or chemical or mechanical abuse. Tackle these using the appropriate herbal solutions and paying special attention to the do's and don'ts under the 'Hair Care' section in this chapter. Chapter 8 will help with advice on how to tackle stress. Poor circulation can be helped by baths and massage (see Chapter 5) and appropriate exercise.

Falling Hair

Make a double-strength decoction using a blend of any of the following herbs:

artichoke leaves
jaborandi
lavender
lime blossom
maidenhair fern
marigold
nasturtium
nettle
quince blossom
rosemary
southernwood
thyme
vine leaves
watercress
willow leaves

Allow to cool. Strain. To a litre of herbal infusion add 120 ml (4 fl oz) of vodka. Dab this liberally into the roots of the hair every day. Do not massage, which will only encourage hair to fall out. The vodka will help to preserve the mixture which should last for at least two months.

To Thicken Hair and Encourage Growth

½ kg (1 lb) honey

250 ml (8 fl oz) almond oil

60 g (2 oz) chamomile for fair hair
or
60 g (2 oz) marjoram for dark hair

Put all the ingredients in a wide-necked jar. Stir, cover and leave to macerate for a week. Strain. Shake well. Section the hair and rub this mixture into the scalp. Cover with a plastic shower cap. Leave on for half an hour. Shampoo out. Use a raspberry leaf conditioning rinse which will help restore the hair to its natural acid balance of about pH-6. There should be enough of this mixture to last for four or five applications as you need only rub it into the scalp.

Dandruff

Dandruff ranges from the dry, flaky, itching kind to redness and inflammation of the scalp. Cider vinegar will greatly relieve the itching but if dandruff has got so bad it is causing inflammation and scabbing consult a trichologist or a dermatologist.

Herbs Which Help Remove Dandruff

sage

boxwood shavings

birch bark

nasturtiums

nettles

rosemary

scabious (use the whole herb including the root)

witchhazel bark

Macerate one or a blend of any of these herbs using 30 g (1 oz) and enough cider vinegar to barely cover. Use fresh herbs as far as possible. Leave the jar tightly stoppered for two weeks. Strain. Section the hair. Soak a pad of gauze in the herbal vinegar and rub it all over the scalp. Let it dry. Brush the hair thoroughly. Rinse well with plain water. Now massage the scalp but do not shampoo. Use this treatment once every two weeks and wash the hair in the interim using a castile-based herbal shampoo containing any of the herbs above.

Alternative Methods of Treating Dandruff

The hot herbal oil treatment. This should not be used on excessively oily hair.

Steer clear of too much alcohol and spicy foods. Never use hairspray, avoid hot dryers and spiky rollers and do not back-comb the hair.

To Stop Freshly Curled Hair Straightening Out

Use rosemary shampoo or a rosemary conditioning rinse.

Natural Hair Setters

Freshly squeezed lemon juice.

Flat beer.

Milk. People with dry hair should use fresh milk, those with oily hair should use powdered skimmed milk made up with water and with a teaspoon of sea salt dissolved in it.

Beaten up egg white.

2 tbsp quince seed

2 litres (3½ pints) rosemary infusion for dark hair
or

2 litres (3½ pints) chamomile infusion for fair hair

2 tbsp rum (white or dark, depending on your hair colour)

6 drops essential oil (rosemary or chamomile, depending on your hair type)

Simmer the quince seed in the herbal infusion until it begins to thicken. Strain out the herbs and seed, mashing the residue well down into the sieve with a wooden spoon. Dissolve the essential oil in the rum. Mix the two lotions together. Save what you do not use in a sterilized bottle. The rum will help to preserve the mixture for a few weeks.

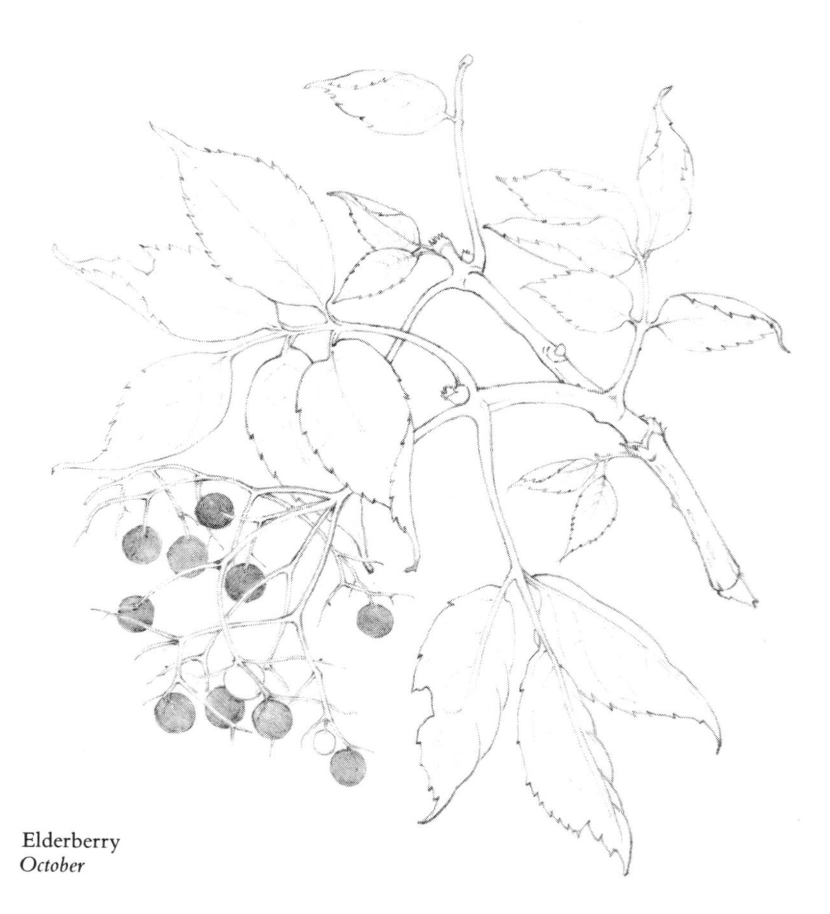

Elderberry
October

Herbal Hair Colouring

Always remember that herbal hair colouring is decidedly unpredictable on hair that has been tampered with chemically, so if you have just had a perm or had your hair dyed only a few weeks ago let the colour or the perm grow out. The nice thing about herbal hair colouring is that it conditions the hair at the same time, improving the texture, giving it body and making it shine. It also develops more slowly than chemical colouring. You may need three or even four applications to see its full effects. Nor will herbal hair colouring change you from a brunette to a blonde. It is much more subtle than that. If you start with a head of raven black hair you can highlight its sheen, giving it plummy overtones with elderberries. On the other hand, if you try to use elderberries on blonde hair you will come out looking a mess – oddly purple and unreal. So be sensible about it. Use red hibiscus to bring out the rosewood undertones, or privet or marigold to bring out the coppery red highlights.

I have starred the herbs which produce the strongest results in their colour change. Use rubber gloves to protect your hands from staining when using these particular herbs. Make a double-strength decoction, not an infusion, of any of the herbs using 60 g (2 oz) to a litre (1¾ pints) of water and boiling in a covered enamel saucepan for fifteen minutes. Keep covered and allow to cool. Strain and then keep pouring the decoction through your hair until your arms get tired. Take special care not to rub the colouring into the scalp, otherwise the stronger colourings will stain the skin. Rinse lightly and towel dry, using an old towel which you do not mind staining, as some of the colouring will inevitably rub off on the towel.

A word of warning about henna. If you have never tried it before I would suggest you seek the professional expertise of a hairdresser as it is very strong and results can prove unpredictable if applied badly by amateur hands. Watch what is being done very closely. Don't be afraid to ask lots of questions so you can use it confidently yourself next time around.

To Lighten Fair or Light Brown Hair

broom flowers
chamomile
*great mullein flowers
*privet
quassia bark
*rhubarb root

To Redden Hair

*alkanet root
cloves
*henna
marigolds
radish root
*red hibiscus
*red oak bark
*red sandalwood
saffron

To Darken Hair

crimson poppies
*green outer shells of unripe walnuts
*ivy berries
raspberry leaves
sage
vinc leaves

To Turn Hair Raven Black

*elderberries

*Indigo leaves used by themselves will produce a violet-blue colour, but mixing with equal quantities of henna will ensure a raven black colour

To Darken Grey Hair

artichoke leaves
betony
marjoram

Alternatively, try thinly slicing the peel of three green oranges and steeping for at least three months in just enough polyunsaturated oil to cover. Strain out the peel and comb the oil through the hair. Leave it on for half an hour and shampoo it out using at least two shampoos to get rid of the oil. This is an Arab remedy for covering up grey hair.

The following old recipe to lighten all hair colours is also most effective but miss out the alum which is included to act as a fixative but which also dries out the hair. Substitute chamomile for turmeric which tends to turn the hair a dull khaki shade. Chamomile will make the hair more golden or brighten the highlights in dark hair.

To make the Hair fair and beautiful

'Cleanse it from Dust, by washing it in Rose-Vinegar, then boil an Ounce of Tumerick, the like quantity of Rhubarb, with the leaves of Bay-tree cut small, to the Quantity of a handful, boiled in a Quart of Water, wherein half a Pound of Allum has been dissolved; and by often washing your Head with the Decoction, it will make your Hair fair and lovely, unless it be Red or exceeding Black.'

John Shirley, *The Accomplished Ladies Rich Closet of Rarities, of The Ingenious Gentlewoman and Servant – Maid's Delightful Companion*, 1715

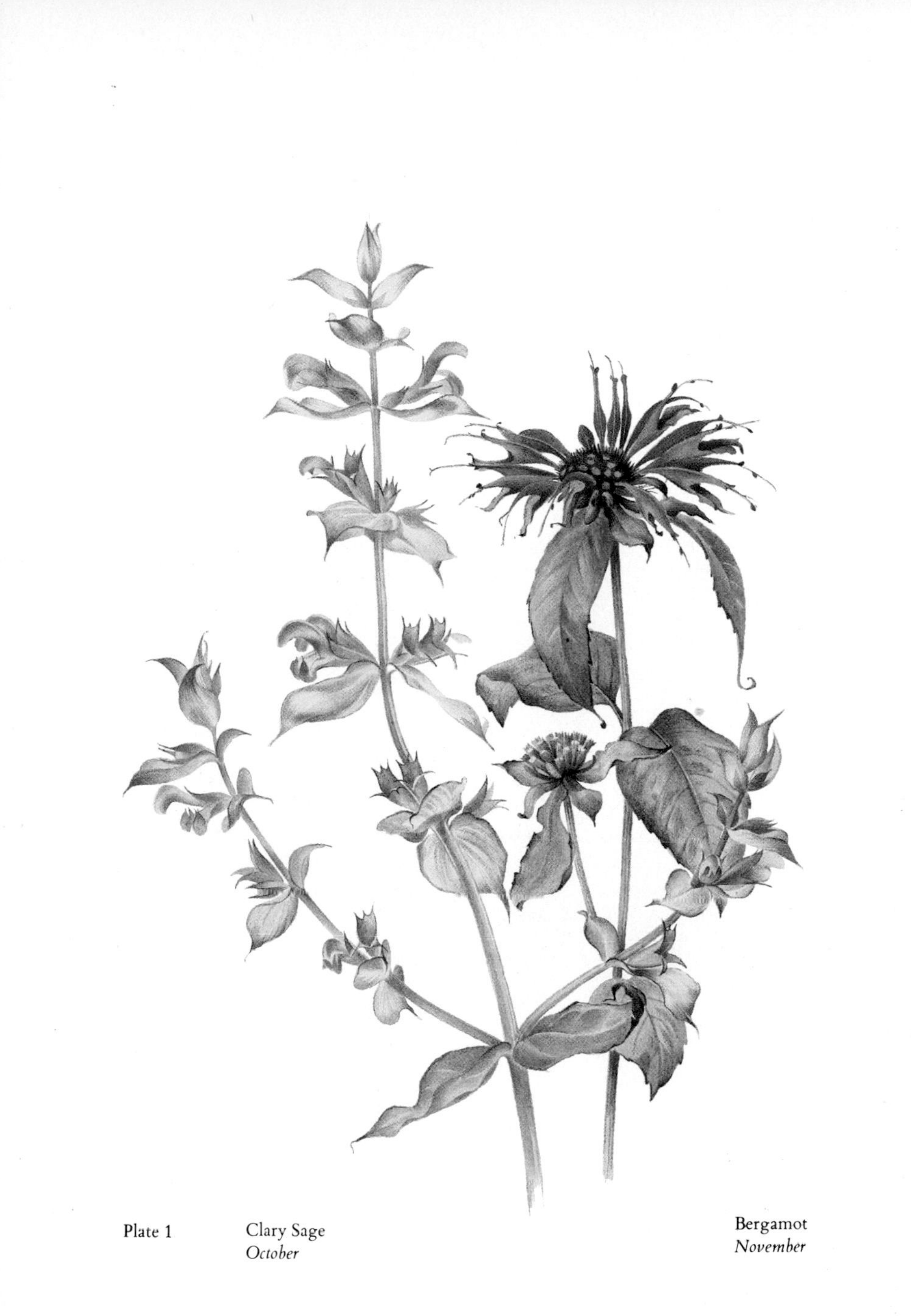

Plate 1 — Clary Sage *October* — Bergamot *November*

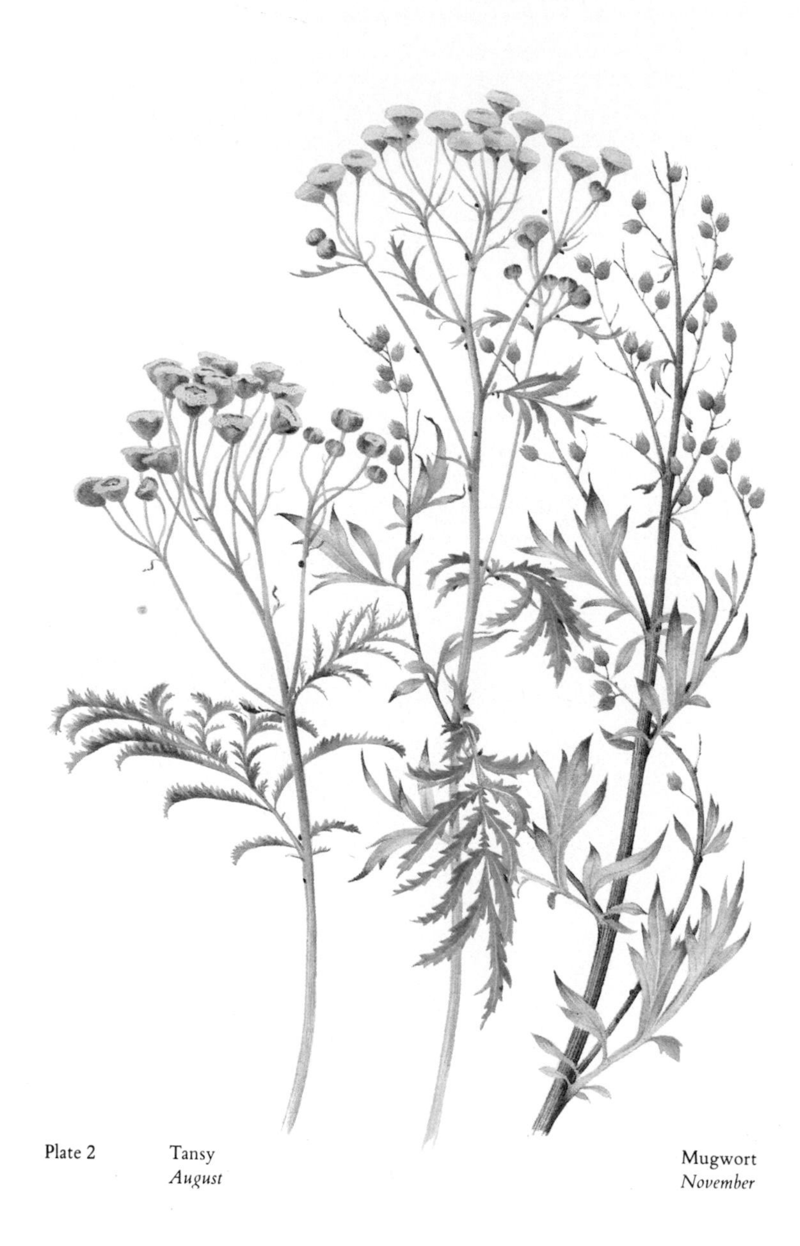

Plate 2 Tansy *August* Mugwort *November*

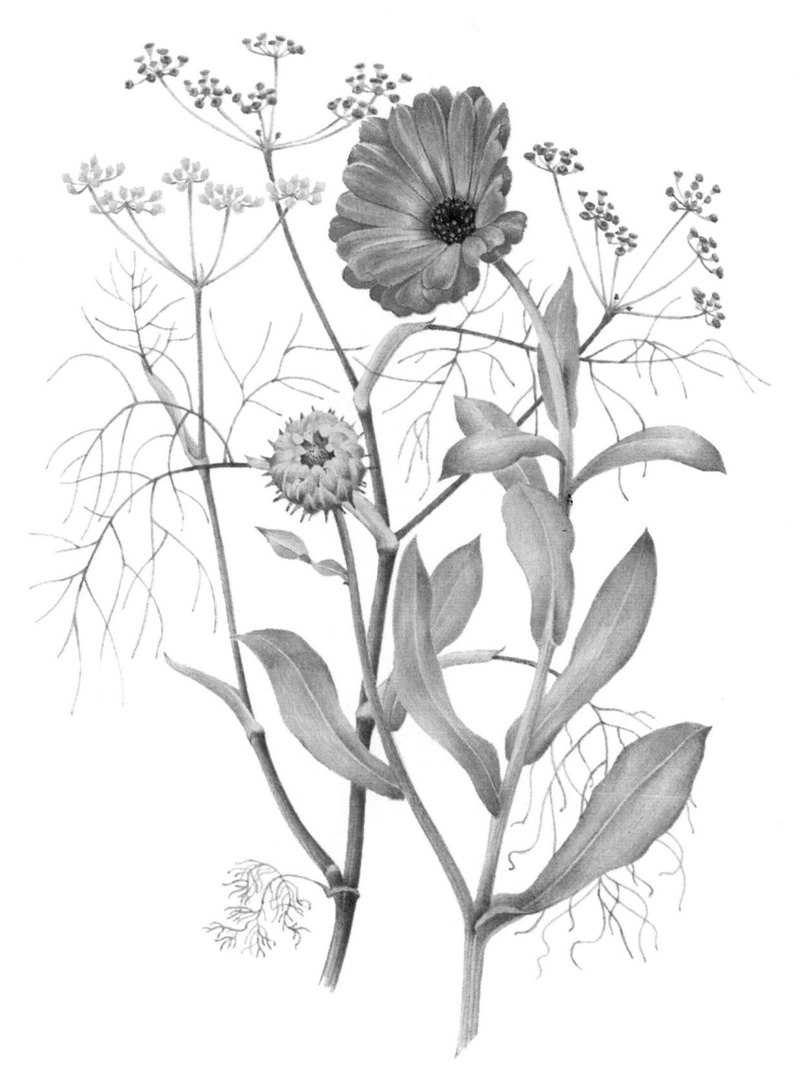

Plate 3 Fennel *October* Marigold *October*

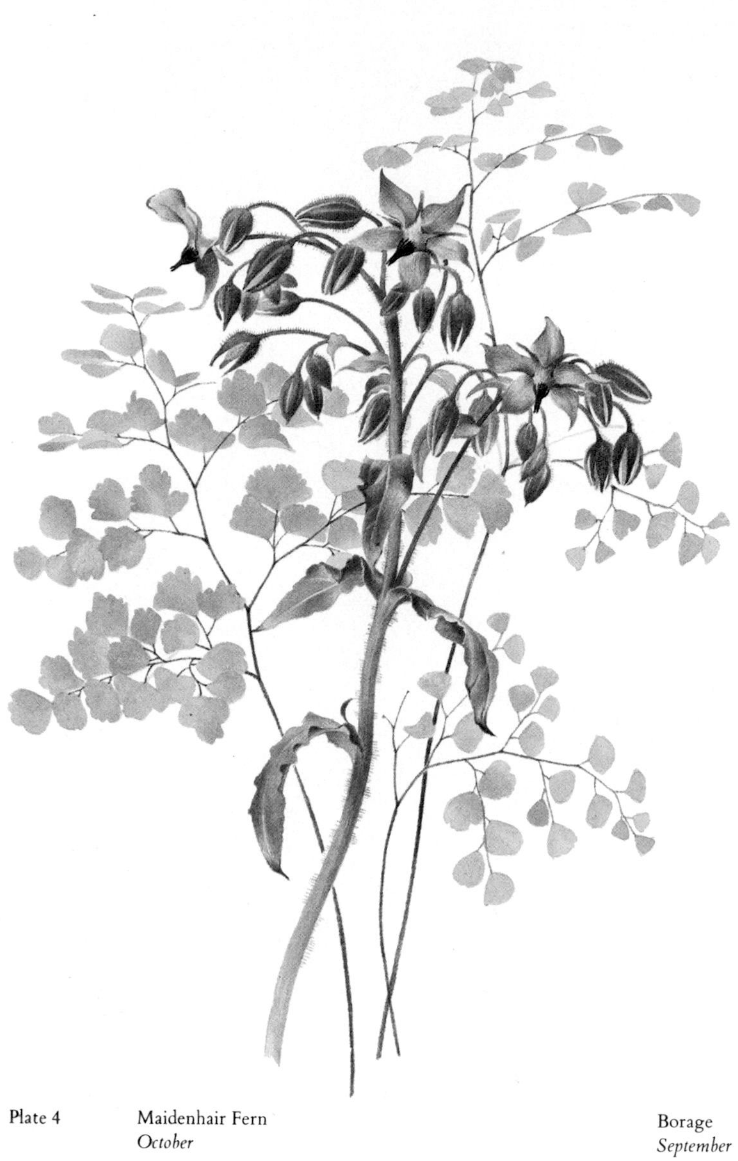

Plate 4 Maidenhair Fern *October* Borage *September*

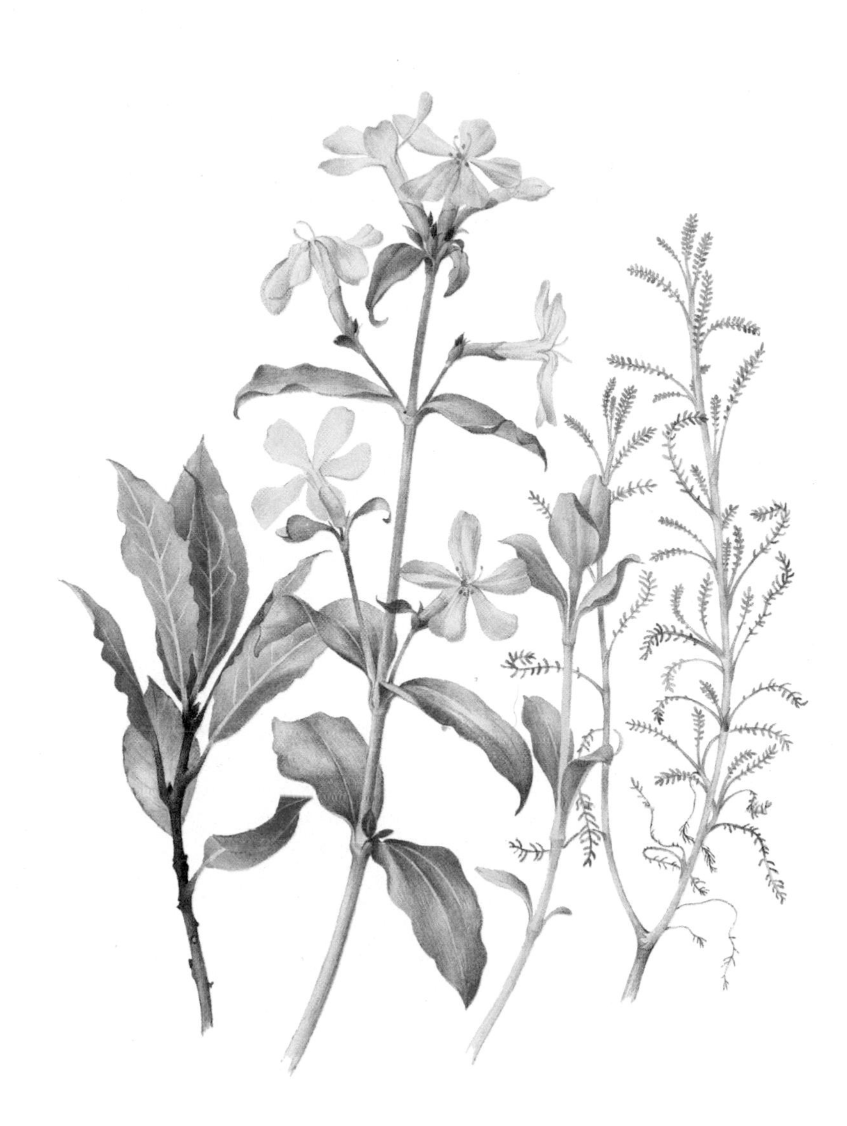

Plate 5 Bay Leaf *November* Soapwort *November* Cotton Lavender *November*

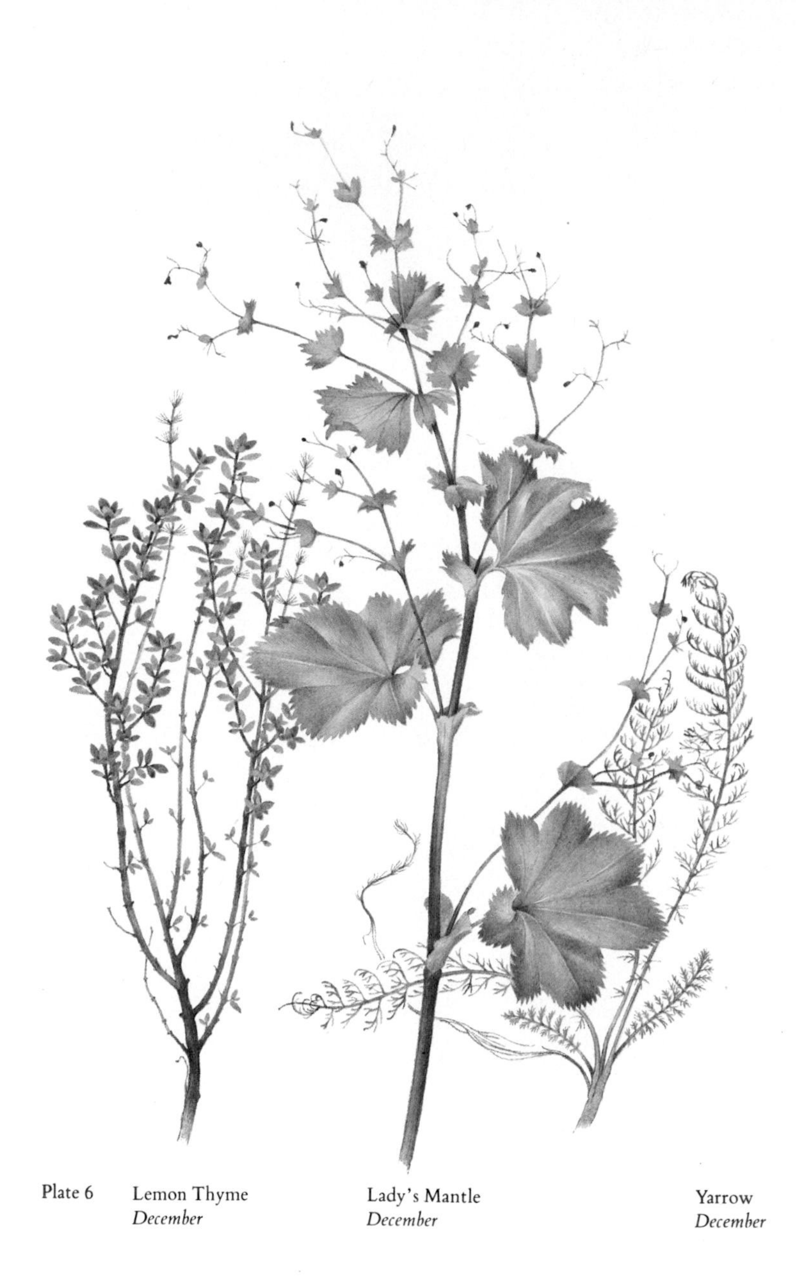

Plate 6 Lemon Thyme *December* Lady's Mantle *December* Yarrow *December*

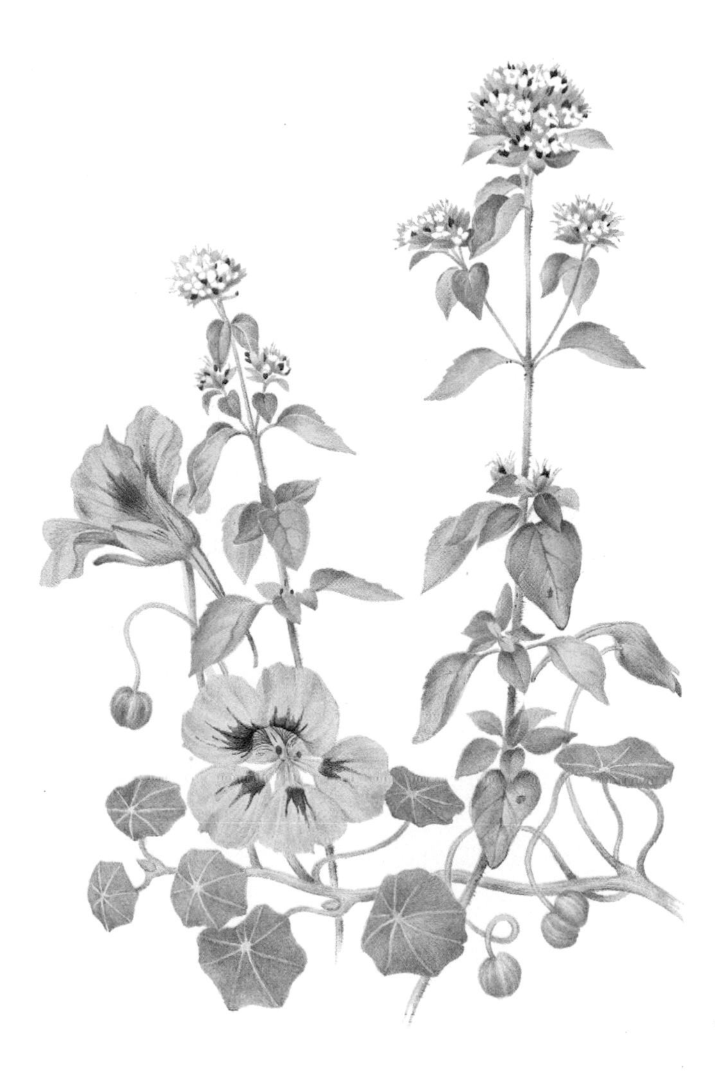

Plate 7 Nasturtium
October

Wild Marjoram
September

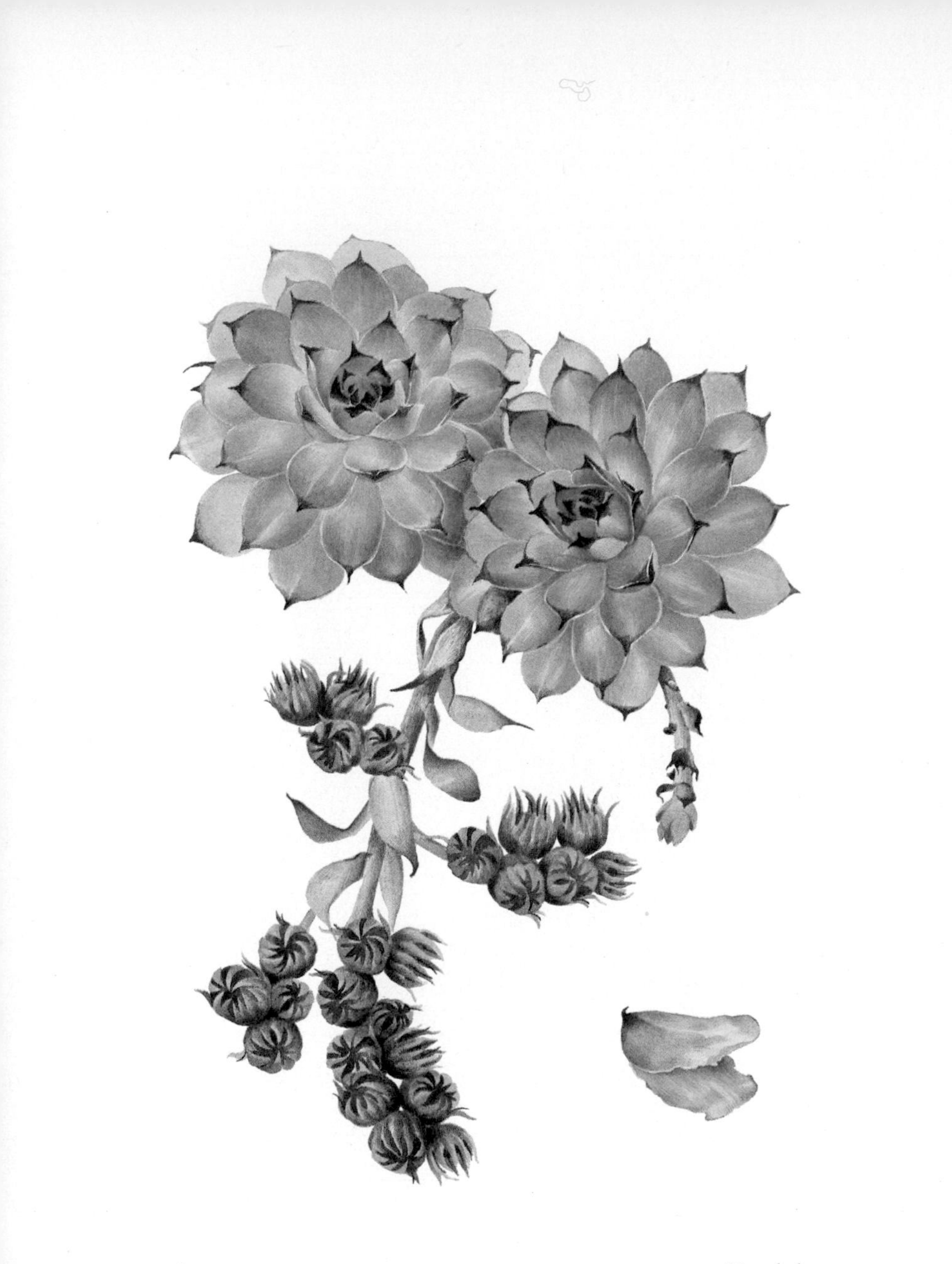

Plate 8

Houseleek
August

Chapter 4

Skin and Hair Care for Men

Unhappily, until some ten or fifteen years ago most men were deliberately brought up not to look in mirrors. Taking grooming seriously was considered the height of vanity and most men scraped by happy with mother's sublime convictions that cleanliness is next to godliness and fresh underwear might be just as well in case they got hit by a bus. A willingness to try even the most unlikely sounding methods to enhance looks was considered an exclusively feminine province. Gradually these double standards have crumbled, and grooming for men has become big business. A sublime disregard for the state of a man's hair, skin and body is no longer considered masculine.

Good grooming is not an unnecessary vanity, nor need it be time-consuming. The advice in this book applies just as much to men as it does to women. Skin, hair, eyes, nails and teeth do not recognize gender. Remember, too, stress and tension take their toll on the body just as much as over-indulgence in drugs, alcohol or tobacco, or food. I am not asking you to become a saint nor, for that matter, a hermit. I have been known to smoke occasionally, to indulge in alcohol to excess and to eat more than one cream cake at a sitting. Life is for living and I have no pretensions towards being a probation officer – or a saint. As far as over-indulgence in any sphere is concerned the Danish proverb 'enough is a great wealth' seems to be a fairly sound maxim to follow. You may not want to go as far as changing the colour of your hair but you will want to keep it clean and in good condition. A good conditioning herbal treatment once or twice a week should make the use of any other hairdressing aids unnecessary.

One of the problems that seems to preoccupy many men is a

receding hairline. A good haircut helps, for it can redirect the eye away from the bald areas to what hair there is. The alternative to camouflage is the really radical step of shaving it all off, which looks deliberate and expresses a lot of self-confidence. Taking this tack is not as crazy as it sounds. Some men look terrific bald – Yul Brynner and Telly Savalas to name but two. Of course, men not blessed with good-shaped craniums don't, but if your move to total baldness proves disastrous, don't worry; the hair you have will always grow back again. Head shaving should be carried out daily to avoid cranial five o'clock shadow. Either way no man should ever allow his baldness to become an obsession. If a man is psychologically unable to handle balding he can always investigate the possibility of using toupées, hair weaving or hair implantation. I need hardly add that he should go to the best, the most reputable and the most experienced firms who employ doctors with appropriate medical qualifications. Some firms do not.

As with all problems prevention is better than cure and herbs to help hair growth and prevent falling hair are listed on pp. 104–106.

Other Tips

Boil 30 g (1 oz) marshmallow roots or maidenhair fern spores in half a litre (1 pint) of white wine in a closely covered enamel saucepan for ten minutes. Allow to cool, still covered. Strain and use as a scalp massage daily.

Grind 30 g (1 oz) parsley seeds finely in a liquidizer. Apply the powder to the scalp once a month. Leave on overnight and brush out the next morning.

Make a double-strength decoction of any of the herbs below; cover and allow to cool for 24 hours before straining. Use it daily, dipping your comb into the decoction and combing your hair gently first in the wrong direction and then back in the right one. Use a comb with rounded, broadly spaced teeth.

- artichoke leaves
- boxwood shavings
- elm tree root
- hemp tops
- jaborandi
- nettles
- rosemary
- southernwood
- tendrils of vines
- willow leaves

If Hair, that comely Ornament of your Sex, be wanting, to recover it
'Take the Ashes of Hyssop, the Juice of Marshmallows, and the Powder of Elicampane-roots, of each an Ounce; boil them in half a Pint of White-wine, with a dram of the Oil of Tartar, till half be consumed, and with the Remainder anoint the bald Place, and the Hair will be restored.'

John Shirley, *The Accomplished Ladies Rich Closet of Rarities, of The Ingenious Gentlewoman and Servant – Maid's Delightful Companion*, 1715

I'm not swearing any of these will work but the fact that they are all old recipes which have been passed down from one generation to another must mean they worked for someone.

Shaving

Pay special attention to the way in which you prepare your skin for shaving. This applies just as much to women who shave their legs or underarms as it does to men. Blade-shavers should choose a really good preshave preparation which will not only wet the beard but lubricate the skin and help the beard swell up, making it easier to cut. Water is the essential prerequisite to a good blade-shave since it reduces beard strength by as much as 60 per cent, so first wash the face with a herbal soap and water to soften the beard and remove any clogging sebaceous oil from the skin. Then rinse and rinse and rinse again with lots of hot water. Now, while your face is still damp, apply a thin film of moisturizer *before* spreading or spraying on the shaving foam. This may sound strange but the moisturizer helps skin lubrication enormously and prevents you from removing the top layer of your skin. The use of a moisturizer at this stage is especially important for dry, tender skins.

If you have used a shaving foam remember it is very drying for the skin because it contains alkaline soap, so splash the face with lots of water until every trace of foam is removed. Now use a herbal aftershave.

Herbal Aftershave

60 ml (2 fl oz) rose water

120 ml (4 fl oz) witchhazel

4 tsp simple tincture of benzoin

12 drops essential oil of bay leaves

2 drops essential oil of rosemary

2 drops essential oil of rose geranium

Pour the benzoin into a large bottle and add the three essential oils. Shake well. The benzoin will dissolve the oils. Now add the flower water and there you have a gentle aftershave with a woody, slightly spicy fragrance. The witchhazel, rosemary and rose geranium are all superb astringents. The rose water and benzoin help to soothe the skin and heal blemishes and the bay leaves are an excellent antiseptic.

Finally, while the skin is still slightly damp with the aftershave, apply a moisturizer appropriate for your skin type. Very dry, sensitive skin types can skip the aftershave altogether and go straight on to the moisturizer. (All the previous information on the skin will help you decide what skin type you have and which moisturizer and herbal soap should be used on it.) A moisturizer is even more essential for a man than for a woman since men do not wear foundation creams or make-up and therefore their skin is always exposed to the elements and to constant atmospheric pollution.

Electric shavers operate most efficiently on a non-oily beard so wash the face thoroughly with herbal soap and water and dry it well before beginning. A pre-electric shaving preparation is a good idea because it helps stiffen the beard and so makes it easier to cut, but because it leaves an oily film on the face it should be removed with a gentle astringent. Carmelite water or the herbal aftershave is ideal for this (for Carmelite water, see p. 202).

Even the most careful shaver occasionally cuts himself. To stem the bleeding crush a couple of fresh yarrow leaves in the palm of your hand and roll these over the cut. This will stem the bleeding instantly and disinfect the wound. Or dab the cut with witchhazel. It stings, but not half as badly as the strong alcohol-based aftershaves available on the market.

If all the advice on shaving is wasted on you because you have a beard, try conditioning your beard with a few drops of essential oil of basil, sage or marjoram if it is a dark beard or with essential oil of chamomile or St John's wort if it is fair or red. Put three drops of the appropriate essential oil into the palm of your hand, rub the palms together to spread it and then rub the tips of a natural bristle brush over the hands so that they pick up the oil. Now brush the beard. All these oils will stimulate growth, complement the colour of your beard and leave it feeling glossy and well-groomed as well as smelling delightful.

Men with oily or sallow skins may like to try an exfoliant face mask monthly in the privacy of their bathrooms. An exfoliant mask should never be used on a freshly shaved skin. Night-time is the right time for this operation. Advice on natural deodorants and skin problems like acne and eczema can be found in Chapter 7. Advice on hair care can be found in Chapter 3. Read Chapter 5 on bathing. Remember, the luxury of an extravagant and relaxing bath is not a female prerogative.

Chapter 5
Body Beautiful

The bath is surely one of the most perfect places to indulge in beauty treatments as well as in relaxation and reverie. We are so used to washing ourselves with soap and water we tend to forget that there are many other extremely effective ways of cleansing the body. Eugene Rimmel, writing in 1865, observed that when the British Consul ordered a bath at Berbera he was rubbed down first with dough and then with perfumed oil. The Consul evidently enjoyed the whole operation hugely and attributed the complete absence of any skin diseases among the natives to its use, saying that it also enabled them to endure the cutting desert winds protected only by thin clothing.

Nomadic tribes have been using fumigation to cleanse themselves for thousands of years. Shortage of water in the desert makes this form of bathing a necessity, but it works very effectively not only to clean and tone the skin but to deodorize and disinfect it. First a hole is dug in the ground and into it is put an earthenware pot containing smouldering aromatic herbs. Then the bather squats over the mixture, covering himself and the hole with a thick woollen cloak in order to trap all the rising fumes. After a few minutes perspiration starts to stream off the body. This process is kept up for ten minutes and followed by a brisk rub-down.

In ancient Egypt nobles took a succession of baths daily, beginning with a cold one and graduating to a hot one perfumed with various herbal oils. The Romans raised bathing to an art, turning it into a social event where they could meet and converse with friends, choosing from a whole range of imaginative alternatives – mineral baths, fruit, vegetable, milk and honey baths, the hypocaustum (the predecessor to our modern Turkish baths) and different types of massage with aromatic oils.

When the Romans conquered Britain the indigenous population would have none of their fancy notions about bathing. They continued to use soapwort and willow ash on the rare occasions they bothered to wash themselves. It was left to the Romans to introduce the herbs they used for toiletries, including lavender (the word is derived from the Latin *lavare*, to wash) which they added to their bath water.

When the Roman Empire collapsed the civilized habit of bathing collapsed with it, although there was a brief resurgence of the art when the Crusaders returned from the East, bringing with them much valuable Arabic knowledge about herbs. By the sixteenth century flower waters were enjoying a revival and Elizabethans used to sprinkle their clothes and floors with 'casting' bottles filled with sweet water. Few of them actually ventured as far as bathing although the very wealthy who did so bathed in the most extravagant liquids. For example, Mary Queen of Scots used to bathe in red wine, a habit which forced the Earl of Shrewsbury, her jailer, to ask for an increase in his government allowance to cover the cost of these expensive ablutions. Anne Boleyn, on the other hand, used to bathe in white wine, which prompted an envious courtier to observe sourly, 'You are doubtless familiar with the degrading sycophancy of the English noblemen who filled their glasses from her bath while she was in it, and drank to her health with revolting jests.' Both ladies chose sensibly for their complexions. Mary was dark and red wine is better for darker greasier skins because, being rich in tannin, it makes a good astringent. Anne Boleyn was fair and white wine is good for toning and lightening the skin.

Baths were taken as much for medication as for beautification. Gervase Markham records a bath reputed to help mend broken joints which includes lye (which would have been decidedly detrimental for the skin whatever it may have done to the bones) and plantain, knot grass, wormwood and comfrey. He also lists:

A generall bath for clearing the skin and comforting the body
'Take Rosemary, Fetherfew, Orgaine, Pellitory of the Wall, Fennell, Mallowes, Violet-leaves, and Nettles, boyle all these to-gether, and when it is well sodden put to it two or three gallons of Milke, then let the Party stand or sit in it an houre or two, and when they come out they must go to bed and beware of taking of cold.'

Gervase Markham, *Countrey Contentments*, 1623

The combination of herbs for this purpose is excellent: nettles stimulate the circulation; fennel tones and tightens the skin; violet leaves and oregano are good herbal antiseptics; the mallows are both soothing and healing, and rosemary is

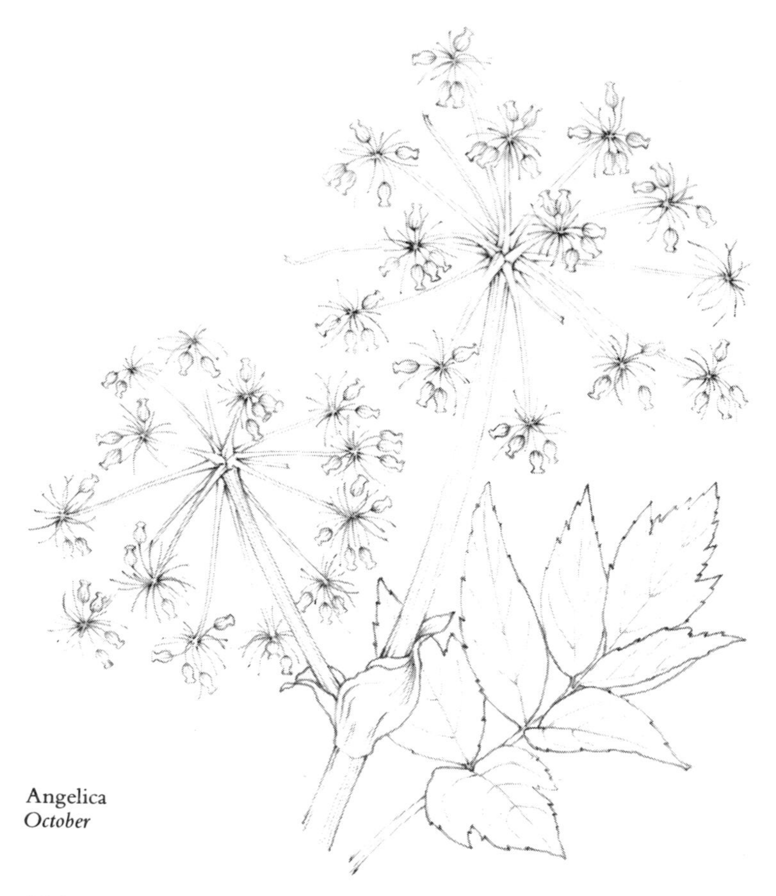

Angelica
October

astringent and helps soothe aching muscles. Milk is, of course, an excellent cleanser, particularly for dry, delicate skins and the cream content in it helps to lubricate the skin: Nero's wife used to bathe in asses' milk, as did Cleopatra; Marie Antoinette used buttermilk compresses to subdue her freckles and lighten her sallow complexion, and Lily Langtry used Jersey cream to preserve her famous complexion.

During the seventeenth century 'sweating houses' were introduced into Britain. The Turks had adopted them from the Romans and after the Great Plague people had rapidly begun to recognize the importance of cleanliness together with the antiseptic value of many herbs. It was not until the nineteenth century that scientists were able to confirm these antiseptic properties. The Pasteur Institute discovered that it was possible to kill tubercular bacilli within twelve hours of exposure to the fumes of essential oil of lavender, and consequently this was used to purify surgical dressings during the First World War when there was a shortage of man-made bactericides. It was discovered that yellow fever micro-organisms were easily killed by essential oils of angelica and thyme, and the latter, which is seven times stronger than carbolic acid, was sprayed on the clothes of soldiers during the Crimean War to protect them from lice and disease.

Sir Hugh Platt describes:

A delicate Stoue to sweat in

'I know that many Gentlewomen, as well for the clearing of their skins, as clensing of their bodies, do now and then delight to sweat. For the which purpose, I have set down this manner following, as the best that euer I obserued: Put into a brasse pot of some good content, such proportion of sweet herbs, and of such kinde as shall be most appropriate for your infirmity, and with some reasonable quantity of water: close the same with an apt couer, and wel-luted with some paste made of flower and whites of Egges: at some part of the couer you must let in a leaden pipe (the entrance where of must be conveyed thorow the side of the chimney) where the pot standeth in a thicke hollow stake of a bathing tub crossed with hoopes, according to the usuall manner, in the top, which you may couer with a sheet of your pleasure. Now, the steam of the pot passing thorow the pipe under the halfe bottome of the bathing tub, which must bee bored full of bigge holes, will breathe so sweet and warm a vapour upon your body, as that (receiving ayre, by holding your head without the tub as you sit therein) you shall sweate most temperately, and continue the same a long time without fainting. And this is performed with a small charcole of fire maintained under the pot for this purpose. Note, that the room would bee close wherein you place your bathing tub, lest any sudden cold should happen to offend you whilst your body is made open and porous to the ayre.'

Delightes for Ladies, 1594

Church dogma had ruled from the fourteenth century that anything concerned with nudity was lewd so Marie Antoinette was taught to bathe under the cumbersome folds of a flannel nightshirt and Louis XIV went one better and boasted that he had never had a bath in his life.

It was not until the nineteenth century that bathing was accepted by all strata of society and even then it was done in the stoic belief that cleanliness was next to godliness rather than for pure pleasure. However, the official church's attitude to nudity persisted: missionaries in the United States were appalled to see members of the Cheyenne tribe bathing in freezing cold rivers. It wasn't the coldness but the nakedness that bothered them. Consequently, the Cheyennes were forced to give up this habit, but until they did so they enjoyed exceptionally good health.

Salt baths, which became popular in Britain with the advent of the bathing machine, were taken in much the same prudish spirit. Layers of clothing were taken off and replaced by voluminous garments hiding every part of the body except the hands, feet and face. The bathing machine was then towed out by a horse to the sea's edge and ladies would descend the ladder and enjoy a brief and very restrictive dip (because of their water-logged garments).

Happily, most of us now acknowledge that bathing can be fun as well as relaxing, hydrating, stimulating, depurative and, of course, cleansing, depending on what you put in the bath and what you take with it. The environment in which you bathe is very important. Leafy green plants, especially ferns, which flourish in the moist, rather dark atmosphere of a bathroom, breathe in stale carbon dioxide and breathe out oxygen, which is quite important in what is usually one of the smallest, least-ventilated rooms in the house. Naked electric light bulbs are not conducive to drifting and dreaming: replace them with shaded lights or candles – perfumed ones are lovely – which should be firmly wedged so that they do not topple over and burn the house down. Soft music also helps, especially if it comes from a radio – this will save you from having to tear yourself away from your reveries to turn over the record. It should go without saying that you should never tamper with electrical equipment in the bath. Have all the bathing equipment you need within easy reach.

Bath Water Temperature

The temperature of your bath water is important. Avoid extremely hot water, which only saps your energy and is bad for the skin, encouraging redness, blotchiness and thread veins. People who have thin skins, varicose veins, any skin disease or those who are overweight or suffer from a heart condition, asthma or hay fever should avoid very hot baths. Bath water should generally be comfortably warm and on very hot days you are better off taking a long soak in a tepid bath, however strong the temptation to lie in a cold one. The tepid water will help dilate your blood vessels so your body can release all its trapped heat. Cold water will only provide temporary relief. After a tepid bath do not aggravate the problem by drying yourself briskly with a towel, simply get out, lie on a towel and air dry.

Herbal Wine Rubs

Enjoy an abbreviated wine bath using the stand up sponge method. Choose red or white wine depending on your skin type. Macerate a combination of the appropriate herbs for your skin (for a list of herbs, see p. 63, and for how to make a wine maceration, see p. 30).

2 cups herbal wine

1 cup coarse sea salt

60 g (2 oz) camphor

Place all the ingredients in a two-litre (half-gallon) bottle and top up with boiling water. Cap and shake vigorously. Allow the mixture to cool to room temperature. Stand in a tub and dip a thick soft cloth in a bowl of the mixture. Gently rub it all over the body, except for the nipples and genital area. Rub yourself dry with a soft towel. This is a variation on the '*eau sédative*' used by Sarah Bernhardt. It is remarkably effective, removing all aches and general fatigue, boosting the circulation and instilling a sense of calm. Best used on those awful days when everyone seems to have been gunning for you since sunrise.

Make up this wine rub freshly each time you use it. The herbal wine most suitable for your skin type will have to be made up in advance, of course, but since herbal wine is so versatile it is always advisable to have a bottle of it handy for toning and for hair rinses.

Isadora Duncan used to keep her skin soft and supple with a daily salt rub. It is messy, so is best carried out standing in the bath or shower, but extremely effective.

Salt Rub

1 tsp coarse sea salt

1 tsp any vegetable oil

2 drops essential oil of your choice

Mix all these together in the palm of your hand. Hop into the tub and rub yourself vigorously with small, circular movements avoiding any delicate areas: you will see dark rolls of dead grey skin peeling off. Rinse yourself with a shower. Pat dry. Your skin will be positively glowing and will feel very soft and supple. If you have chosen your essential oil wisely it will also smell lovely too.

I have never found the modern equivalent of the milk bath – a packet of dried milk – as effective as the real thing. The effects of a few spoonfuls of dried milk are very limited as the milk is so diluted but few of us can afford Poppaea's solution of forty asses which kept her well supplied with the material she needed for her milk bath. A milk sponge bath is a viable modern alternative and leaves your skin feeling silky and smooth.

Milk Sponge Bath

2 cups full cream milk

1 tbsp clear honey

juice of 2 oranges, strained

Warm the milk and stir the honey into it until it dissolves. Allow to cool to tepid, then add the orange juice. Decant into a bowl and sponge this mixture all over your body. Leave it on for fifteen minutes, wrapping yourself in a towel to keep warm once the milk has dried on the skin, then shower off and pat yourself dry.

Oatmeal Rub

2 cups flaky oatmeal

½ cup yoghurt, buttermilk or cream

2 egg yolks

Beat all the ingredients together. Stand in the bath and rub your body with this paste. It may be messy but it revitalizes a dingy sallow skin amazingly quickly.

Nervous Tension Rub

60 g (2 oz) poppy flowers

½ litre (1 pint) water

Make a decoction, boiling in a closely covered enamel saucepan for thirty minutes. Strain. Get someone to rub this water, while it is still warm, if possible, into the small of your back and the area round the neck and shoulders.

Herbal Baths

You can take a herbal bath in various ways:

Add ten drops of any essential oil appropriate for your skin type to the bath water once it has been run.

Take a cup of herbs and simmer them in 2 litres (3½ pints) of water in a covered enamel saucepan for fifteen minutes. Strain the decoction and pour it into your bath water. Tie up the residue in a muslin square to which you have added a handful of oatmeal, almond meal or bran (a strong rubber band helps here). Use this bag as a flannel while you are in the bath.

Herbal decoctions can, of course, be made up in advance and stored in the refrigerator for up to three days. Use a large sterilized glass or earthenware container and cover the top with a piece of muslin or absorbent kitchen paper towel. Do not use cling film which will only encourage the decoction to ferment.

When using a refrigerated decoction remember to draw a bath which is a little hotter than usual as once you add the ice cold decoction it will lower the temperature noticeably. Do not attempt to keep the herb residue for use in a muslin square for more than twenty-four hours as the herbs will start to rot fairly quickly. Throw the strained herbs on the compost heap instead.

Tie a generous handful of herbs in a muslin square and throw this in the water while it is running. Again, use this as your flannel.

If you are feeling particularly rushed or lazy throw a few herbal tea bags in the water while it is running. These are too fragile to be used as a flannel.

The one thing you really should not do is throw a handful of herbs straight into the water with delighted abandon. Your delight will soon evaporate when the drain blocks up and you have to spend hours picking the leafy residue off your body.

Cleansing Herbal Bath

A cupful made up of equal quantities of the following herbs:

borage

lemon balm

meadowsweet

rose petals

sage

Add the herbs to 2 litres (3½ pints) of water in a covered enamel saucepan and simmer for fifteen minutes. Strain and pour into warm bath water.

Soothing Herbal Bath

This is especially good for people with raw itchy skin. A cupful made up of equal quantities of:

comfrey

houseleek

lady's mantle

marshmallow

Put the herbs in a large square of muslin and secure with a rubber band. Throw the bundle into a bathful of warm water and leave to macerate for five minutes. Squeeze the bag well. Remove from the bath water and add a cupful of cider vinegar to the water, together with three tablespoons of any herbal syrup.

Prickly Heat Bath

1 cup comfrey

1 cup houseleek

2 litres (3½ pints) water

Simmer the herbs in the water in an enamel saucepan for thirty minutes. Strain. Pour into the bath water and add a tablespoon of honey and a cupful of laundry starch. Make sure the water is barely lukewarm.

Stimulating Bath

A cupful made up of equal quantities of:

lavender

lemon thyme

marjoram

peppermint

rosemary

Follow instructions for cleansing bath on p. 127. This bath can also be enjoyed using 60 g (2 oz) of dried herbs to the same quantity of water.

An Extra-special Stimulating Bath

½ cup pine needles

1 cup nettles

2½ litres (4½ pints) water

4 drops essential oil of basil

Boil up the pine needles in half a litre (1 pint) of water in an open enamel saucepan for forty-five minutes. Strain out the pine needles and continue to boil the decoction until it is just beginning to turn syrupy. Infuse the nettles for half an hour in the remaining 2 litres (3½ pints) of water while your pine needles are bubbling away. Strain out the nettles. Pour the infusion and the decoction into the bath. Add the essential oil of basil. This will really get your skin tingling. Dried nettles can be substituted for fresh, in which case use 30 g (1 oz). Use the same quantity of pine needles whether fresh or dried.

Deodorant Bath

1 cup parsley

1 cup cleavers (leaves and flowers if possible)

1 cup lovage (leaves and stalks)

2 litres (3½ pints) water

Boil all the herbs in the water in a closely covered enamel saucepan for half an hour. Strain. Save a cupful to splash liberally over the areas which tend to perspire the most – the armpits, behind the knees and feet and under the breasts – and pour the rest into lukewarm bath water. Do not use this mixture to deodorize the genital area as it may cause irritation. Refer instead to the section on douches on p. 142.

Tranquillizing Bath

3 tbsp linden blossom

3 tbsp chamomile

3 tbsp violets

3 tbsp cowslips

1 tbsp great mullein (flowers)

3 tbsp woodruff

1 tbsp mistletoe (leaves)

3 litres (5¼ pints) water

3 tbsp vervain or valerian (root)

Make a decoction and boil for twenty minutes. Strain. Pour into a lukewarm bath. Add two tablespoons of herbal syrup and stir this well into the water until it dissolves. Relax. Have a long soak. Sip a cup of chamomile or linden tea while you do so (see also chamomile bath, p. 203). If fresh herbs are out of season use dried ones, substituting teaspoon for tablespoon

Vervain
November

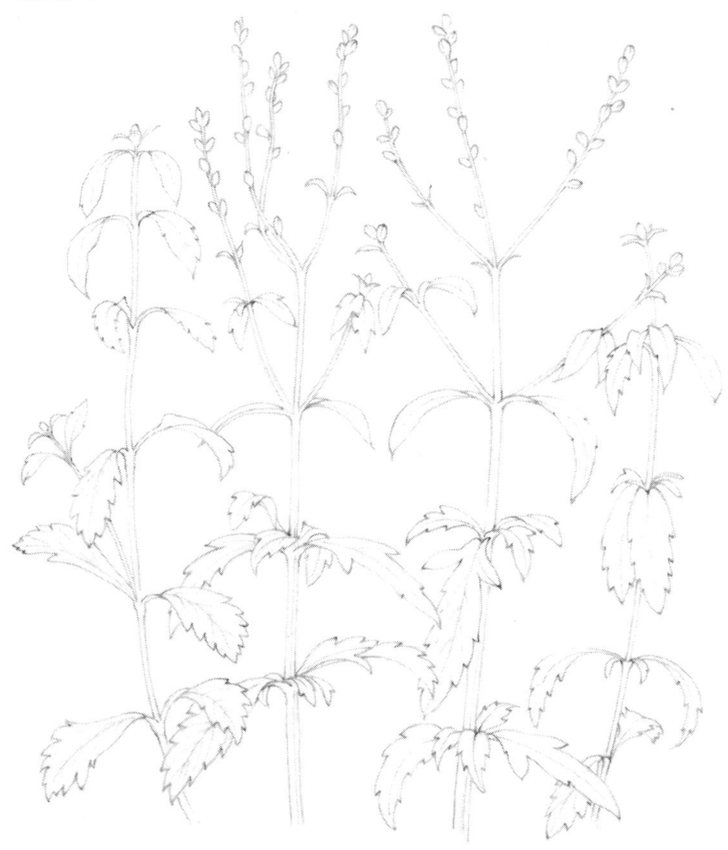

measurements throughout, and using the same quantity of water.

To Alleviate Aches and Pains

A cupful of equal parts of the following herbs:

agrimony	burdock

comfrey

mugwort

sage

St John's wort

1 litre (1¾ pints) water

1 tbsp Epsom salts

Make a decoction and boil for twenty minutes. Strain. Add to the bath water together with the Epsom salts.

Strengthening Bath

This is not supposed to increase your biceps. It will, however, strengthen the skin on the body, and so is especially good for people with thin, delicate skins. It has the added bonus of stopping a cold dead in its tracks if you are just beginning to feel feverish and your temperature is rising. As a skin-strengthening treatment this bath should be taken three times a week for several months.

3 tbsp salad burnet

3 tbsp thyme

3 tbsp rosemary

2 tbsp basil

3 tbsp marjoram

3 tbsp hyssop

3 litres (5¼ pints) water

4 tbsp fennel (seed, bruised with a pestle and mortar)

Make a decoction, boiling in a closely covered enamel saucepan for thirty minutes. Strain and add to the bath with two tablespoons of honey and a teaspoon of wheatgerm oil.

Cold-relieving Bath

2 tbsp chamomile

2 tbsp linden blossom

2 tbsp elderflowers

2 tbsp borage (leaves)

2 tbsp burdock

1½ litres (2¾ pints) water

Make a decoction of the herbs, boiling in a closely covered enamel saucepan for twenty minutes. Strain. Add to fairly hot bath water. You will probably feel far too fragile to rub yourself with anything, but if you can, use the residue of herbs tied in a muslin bag as a flannel. Lie in the bath and sip a cup of herbal tea made from equal parts of chamomile, linden and elderflowers and sweeten with a teaspoon of honey. Pat yourself dry, do not rub. Hop into bed and sweat it out. Dried herbs can be substituted for fresh, in which case change the tablespoon measurements to teaspoons and use the same quantity of water.

Aphrodisiac Bath

The best aphrodisiac is obviously the person you are bathing with, but this will help.

2 tbsp nasturtium leaves

2 tbsp rose petals

1 tbsp bay leaves

2 tbsp rosemary

1 tbsp dried ginseng root

2 tbsp rocket (leaves)

2 tbsp honeysuckle

2 litres ($3\frac{1}{2}$ pints) water

4 drops neroli oil (oil made from orange blossom)

Make a decoction of all the herbs and simmer them in a closely covered enamel saucepan for fifteen minutes. Strain. Add to the bath water. This combination of herbs has a lovely sweet woody smell. Swish in the neroli oil. The rest is up to you! (Suppliers of neroli oil and many other essential oils are listed in Appendix II.)

Bath Oils

Store all bath and massage oils in opaque bottles with narrow openings. This will prevent you from pouring a great dollop into your bath water or your hand by accident. You can fix the perfume of any of your bath oils with a few drops of essential oil of sandalwood. All oils can be made up ahead of time and will keep indefinitely. Use only natural oils for all bath and massage oils. Mineral oils, for reasons outlined on p. 55, should not be used.

Floating Bath Oils

These will help dry, scaling and itching skin by protecting and lubricating it. They are easily made, using any natural oil mixed with an essential oil of your choice. The amount you add depends on the quality of the essential oil and on how strong you want the bath oil to smell, but as a general guide ten drops of any essential oil to a tablespoon of vegetable or nut oil is about right. If you use much more than this the essential oil can irritate the skin. This is particularly true of the more stimulating essential oils – basil, all the mints, bergamot, hyssop, juniper, thyme and rosemary. Add a little wheatgerm oil to your natural oil base and use about one tablespoon of bath oil at a time, adding it to the water after it has been drawn. If you add it while the water is running much of the fragrance will evaporate before you get into the bath. Lie in the bath and massage yourself by scooping up handfuls of oily water and rubbing them into the skin.

One of the disadvantages of this type of bath oil is that it leaves a nasty greasy ring round the tub and the last thing you want to do is emerge feeling smooth and fragrant, then have to get to work with the scouring powder. The other disadvantage is that it makes the tub somewhat slippery so be careful as you get in and out. Nevertheless, floating bath oils do leave the skin feeling smooth and well-moisturized, especially if you massage your skin while in the bath.

Dispersing Bath Oils

These neatly circumvent both the disadvantages of floating bath oil. They are based on sulphonated castor oil – oil from the castor plant which has been treated. It is sometimes known as 'Turkey Red' oil and although it looks thick, brown and unpromising it actually dissolves in water. Mix a tablespoon of this oil with six drops of any essential oil of your choice and add it to the bath water. The water may foam slightly at first, but I am sure you will not mind that.

Rich Dispersing Oil

60 g (2 oz) beeswax

30 ml (1 fl oz) sesame oil

90 ml (3 fl oz) almond oil

1½ tsp simple tincture of benzoin

8 drops essential oil of your choice

Melt the beeswax and the sesame and almond oils together. Pour the simple tincture of benzoin into a bottle. Add the essential oil and shake hard. The simple tincture of benzoin will dissolve the oil. Now slowly pour the benzoin mixture into the melted oils stirring hard all the time. The benzoin will give the formula a milky tinge. Add two tablespoons of this to your bath and save the rest for future use in an opaque tightly stoppered bottle.

Massage Oils

These are made in exactly the same way as bath oils. Use only a teaspoon at a time. A little goes a long way. Pay special attention to dry heels, elbows and knees.

Invigorating Massage Oil

1 tbsp almond oil

1 tsp wheatgerm oil

3 drops essential oil of peppermint

3 drops essential oil of bergamot

3 drops essential oil of basil

Erotic Massage Oil (so called because it smells so fantastic)

1 tbsp avocado oil

1 tsp wheatgerm oil

2 drops essential oil of sandalwood

3 drops essential oil of jasmine

3 drops essential oil of rose

Anti-wrinkle Oil

½ tbsp peach kernel oil

½ tbsp wheatgerm oil

3 drops essential oil of fennel

2 drops essential oil of lavender

3 drops essential oil of neroli

This is particularly good for smoothing and toning crepey skin on the neck and for softening wrinkles on the face.

Honey and Almond Body Lotion

50 g (1⅔ oz) anhydrous lanolin

1 tbsp honey

60 ml (2 fl oz) almond oil

30 ml (1 fl oz) wheatgerm oil

60 ml (2 fl oz) orange flower water

3–6 drops essential oil of chamomile

Follow the Basic Lotion Directions on p. 58, stirring the honey into the lanolin once it has melted. This makes a thick lotion which can be used liberally all over the body. It is especially good for application after sunbathing or skiing. This lotion is not suitable for massage as it is absorbed too quickly by the skin but it is an excellent protective moisturizer.

Deodorants

Perspiration is almost odourless. It is only when it is mixed with bacteria that it smells offensive. The most obvious solution to the problem is to wash away the bacteria frequently by bathing, using herbs that deodorize the skin or herbs that smell nice and thus sweeten the body. Clothes are another important factor. Change your clothes often, and wear natural fabrics as much as you can – synthetic ones stop the skin breathing. Fraught emotions also produce perspiration. Normally you sweat several pints a day but this can increase to as many as twenty pints if you are indulging in strenuous physical exercise or are panic-stricken. Worrying about B.O. can make it worse and there you are trapped in a vicious cycle. What can you do about it?

Firstly, apply a deodorant only fifteen or twenty minutes after you have had a bath or shower. You may emerge all sweet and clean but all that heat and moisture will have increased your perspiration level. Give your body time to calm down. Secondly, try a natural deodorant. The underarms can develop a natural immunity to synthetic deodorants which are constantly applied. This is less true of natural deodorants, though you can still alternate natural deodorants and let your body play the guessing game.

Natural Solutions

A double-strength decoction of sage and/or thyme.

Witchhazel diluted 1:2 with purified water.

A decoction of lovage, cleavers and parsley (see p. 27).

Try incorporating sage, lovage and parsley into your daily diet. Eat live yoghurt daily: this will gradually help to change the bacterial colonies in and eventually on your body for the better.

Finely powdered lavender, rose petals, thyme, liquorice root, chamomile and sage can all be mixed into talc 1:3 and used as underarm deodorant powders. Choose the herb you like the smell of best. Lavender, liquorice root, rose petals and sage tend to stain light clothing so be careful.

Begin by using only one of these solutions and see how far they help to solve the problem. You may find incorporating the appropriate herbs and live yoghurt into your diet enough to do the trick. People with a really difficult body odour problem may need to use a daily deodorizing bath, a deodorizing decoction for under the arms and a deodorant powder.

Powders

You can make your own herbal powders by mixing finely powdered and sieved herbs into unscented talcum powder or arrowroot. Alternatively, you can macerate the whole herb of your choice in a box of talcum powder for a few weeks, waiting while the powder absorbs the smell of the herbs, then sifting the herbs out. This method produces a more delicate smelling powder. You can add a few drops of an essential oil of your choice to unscented talc, stir it in well and leave it tightly covered while it is being absorbed. A base of powdered yellow sandalwood or orris root can be used instead of arrowroot or talc but these two ingredients are really only suitable for resilient skins as they are coarse and somewhat gritty and should not be dabbed under arms, breasts or in the genital area.

Prickly Heat Powder

120 g (4 oz) arrowroot

60 g (2 oz) dried chamomile

Pound the chamomile with a pestle and mortar until it is reduced to a fine powder. Mix in the arrowroot then sift the whole mixture through a very fine meshed hair sieve discarding any lumps. Keep in a tightly covered box.

To Make Perfumed Powder
'Take four ounces of Florence Orris, four ounces of dry'd Damask Roses, half an Ounce of Benjamin, a quarter of an Ounce of

Storax,[1] as much of yellow Saunders, half a dram of Cloves,[2] and a little Citron Peel; pound all these in a Mortar to a very fine Powder, put to them five pounds of Starch pounded, mix them well, sift it fine, and keep it dry for use.'

Charles Carter (cook to the Duke of Argyll), *The Compleat City and Country Cook*, 1732

Florence Orris is orris root, Benjamin is benzoin, Saunders is sandalwood. Make sure to use yellow not red sandalwood. Do not use laundry starch unless you want to glue yourself together. Try arrowroot or unscented talc and reduce the quantities appropriately. This makes a lovely spicy powder, though it does need a lot of sifting.

Exotic and Erotic Powder

The smell of this powder is only just this side of heaven. It is a very far cry from the synthetically perfumed gardenia or jasmine talc available commercially.

1 litre (1 quart) of freshly picked gardenias or jasmine flowers

arrowroot to cover

Pick your flowers and measure them out. Do not cram them into the measuring jug which will bruise them. Pack them loosely. Make sure they are water- and insect-free. Lay them in a cardboard box and cover with arrowroot. Close the box tightly and shake it five or six times daily. After three days sift out the flowers. If the perfume is not strong enough for you repeat the whole process using the same powder but fresh flowers. Wildly extravagant but well worth it. If you do not have any gardenia or jasmine flowers you can try the same recipe using the most fragrant roses or scented rose geranium leaves you have. Not as exotic or erotic but special in their own way.

1. Storax is a sweet smelling gum resin extracted from the tree *Styrax officinalis*. I missed out this last ingredient as it is no longer obtainable.
2. About 25 cloves.

Breasts

Breasts may come and go as far as fashion is concerned but there is no doubt about it, they are one of the most pleasing aspects of a woman and the breasts one has should be kept in good shape, which is difficult because the breasts themselves contain no muscles. However, they are supported by the surrounding muscles running into the back, shoulder and chest, so keep these in trim. Stand with your elbows out then press your hands together at waist level as if you were praying in a very upright fashion. Press hard. Count to ten. Relax. Now adopt the same posture but move your hands up to breast level. Repeat. Finally, push your hands straight out in front of you against a wall. Press the wall hard, count to ten, relax. Do this several times and as often as you think of it.

Do not neglect to massage and moisturize your breasts. You should moisturize your breasts whenever you apply a moisturizer to your face and do not miss out the gap in between – your neck, your shoulders and collarbone. Rub in the moisturizer in large rotating circles with your fingers pointed inwards towards the nipple. Start from the outer edge of the breast and work inwards.

Breast Massage Oil

This includes lady's mantle, which has been long valued by the Arabs for all women's complaints. They call it *alkemelych* (alchemy) because of what they believe are its wonder-working powers.

60 ml (2 fl oz) almond oil

60 ml (2 fl oz) wheatgerm oil

20 drops essential oil of lady's mantle

a few drops essential oil of your choice to perfume (optional)

If you miss the perfume out the oil tends to smell slightly chocolatey because of the wheatgerm oil, which is rather pleasant. The lady's mantle oil hardly smells at all. Massage a little of this oil well into the breasts nightly, dabbing off any excess with absorbent tissues.

Breasts, stomach and thighs are the areas which tend to expand rapidly when one puts on weight quickly and the result of the sudden skin stretching can be ugly stretch marks. Adelle Davis, in *Let's Get Well*, records:

A friend who developed severe stretch marks during her first pregnancy stayed on an unusually adequate high-protein diet supplemented with 600 units of vitamin E oil and 300 mls panthothemic acid daily throughout a subsequent pregnancy. Although she gave birth to full-term twins, the stretch marks from the first pregnancy completely disappeared and none formed during the second pregnancy.

This sounds well worth bearing in mind, but if the damage has already been done try the following lotion. Better still, use it regularly morning and evening while you are expanding.

Stretch Mark Lotion for Breasts and Stomach

15 g (½ oz) beeswax

15 g (½ oz) cocoa butter

50 ml (1⅔ fl oz) coconut oil

30 ml (1 fl oz) wheatgerm oil

60 ml (2 fl oz) decoction of lady's mantle and woodruff

3–6 drops essential oil of comfrey

Follow the Basic Lotion Directions, (p. 58).

Add a teaspoon of wheatgerm oil to every bath.

Stretch Mark Erasing Lotion for the Rest of the Body

30 ml (1 fl oz) infusion of borage leaves

60 ml (2 fl oz) rose vinegar

30 g (1 oz) cocoa butter

70 ml (2⅓ fl oz) coconut oil

20 ml (⅔ fl oz or 4 tsp) wheatgerm oil

Pound the borage leaves to a pulp and scrape this into the rose vinegar. Macerate the mixture for a fortnight. Strain it through coffee filter paper. Proceed with the Basic Lotion Directions, (p. 58) using the borage-rose concoction for the water phase. Rub this lotion liberally into the stretch marks twice daily.

Melt a tablespoon of coconut oil until it is liquid and add this to your daily bath.

Should you ever be unfortunate enough to get sunburned nipples try a warm poultice of comfrey applied twice daily. A poultice of yarrow and lady's mantle will help heal cracked and weeping nipples. Sore nipples, usually the result of nursing, can be soothed by massaging in a teaspoon of glycerine or honey mixed with four drops of simple tincture of benzoin.

Sore breasts can be soothed by a daily application of the following poultice:

'Takc a whitc winc and minglc flowcr with it and makc it as thick as boyled thickened milk, then boyle it till it be as thick as hasty pudding bc surc to brcak all ye lumps bcforc you sctt it on ye firc and stir it well while it is on, when it is as thick as you can stirr it, put into a pint of it, a quarter of a pound of bears grease. Stir it well till it is melted then take it off ye fire and put in ye whites of 4 eggs well beaten, It must be a large pint y^t you put there things into you must work ye Eggs till it is as smooth as past, work it at least quarter of an hour.'

Mary Doggett, *Book of Receipts*, 1682

I used cornflour to solve the lump problem and hydrous lanolin instead of bear's grease. Remember to let it cool to blood heat before applying it. A hot poultice is guaranteed to make the problem worse. Best applied while lying in a shallow bath and the residue will wash away obligingly without blocking up the plug hole.

Some old herbals recommended a poultice of mashed cooked turnip to help sore breasts. I have never tried this but it crops up so frequently, our ancestors obviously found it worked.

Douches

Douches, used sensibly and in moderation, are an excellent way to keep the vagina healthy as they cut down on the incidence of vaginitis, which two out of every three women

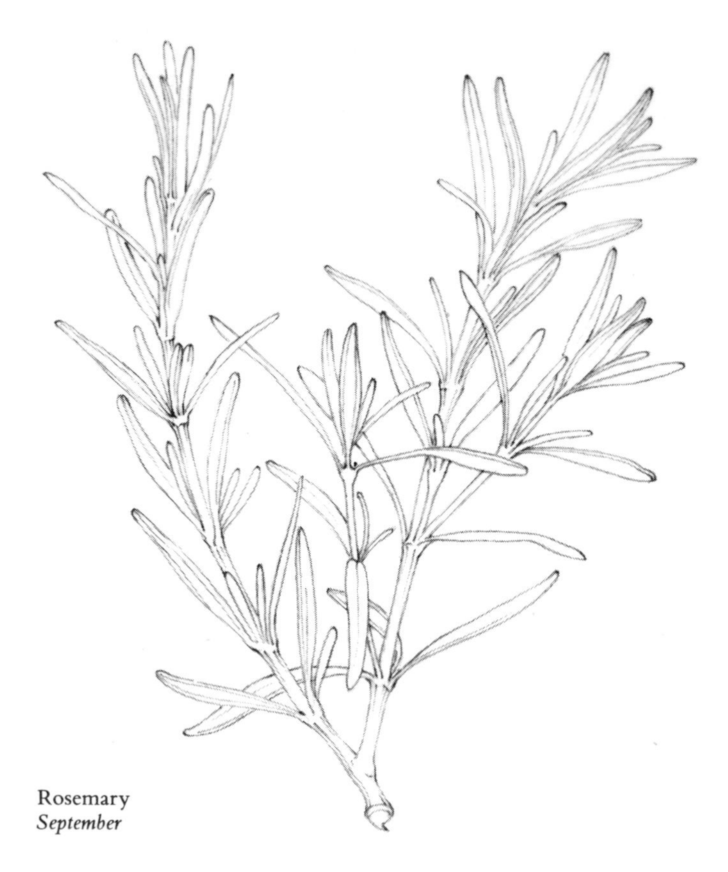

Rosemary
September

suffer from at some time during their lives. Douching seems decidedly unfashionable in Britain as I discovered when I tried to buy a douche bag and syringe. As you will encounter the same problem I have included a list of stockists in Appendix II. Happily, the Continentals and Americans seem more *au fait* with douches.

To take a douche just fill the douche bag with 1¼ litres (2 pints) of water which have been thoroughly boiled and allowed to cool to lukewarm. Add four tablespoons of any of the following douche mixtures, hang the douche bag about a foot above the bath and lie down. Insert the nozzle about 3·5 cm (1½ in.) into your vagina. Release the clamp slowly so that the water does not rush into your vagina, letting it run in and drain out. Gentleness is important because a stream of water that is too forceful can push the water through from the uterus to the fallopian tubes and into the abdominal cavity. Needless to say pregnant women should never douche. Of course you should always remember to keep your douche bag and syringe scrupulously clean. Store it in a plastic bag when it is not in use.

Raspberry Vinegar Douche

1 tbsp rosemary

1 tbsp rose petals

1 tbsp fresh raspberries

2 cups cider vinegar

Pound the herbs. Squash the fruit. Macerate both in the cider vinegar in a closely covered sterilized container for two weeks. Strain the mixture through coffee filter paper. Add four tablespoons to the freshly boiled and cooled water in your douche bag and rebottle the remainder in a sterilized container. The cider vinegar in this douche helps to keep the vagina acid which kills off yeasts, fungi and other harmful organisms. It is only when this balance is upset that some organisms multiply out of all proportion causing yeast and other vaginal infections.

Yeast infections, commonly called thrush, can be helped by this douche and the following one.

Blackberry Douche

1 tbsp blackberry leaves	1 tbsp marshmallow
1 tbsp lavender	1 tbsp sage
1 tbsp daisies	1 litre (1¾ pints) water

Make an infusion. Strain through coffee filter paper and add four tablespoons to your douche bag. Blackberry leaves, lavender and daisies are all especially helpful for thrush, while the marshmallow is soothing and decongestive and the sage acts as a tonic for the uterus.

WARNING. Some people are allergic to a group of plants which includes bergamot, chamomile and daisies. As this is for use in the vagina try a patch test of daisy infusion on your wrist first. If there is any redness or irritation as a result of the test omit the daisies from the douche altogether.

Aphrodisiac Douche

1 tbsp scented geranium	½ tbsp clary sage
1 tbsp violet flowers	½ litre (1 pint) water

Make an infusion and allow to stand for ten minutes. Strain and add six tablespoons to the water in your douche bag. This is so called because it smells and tastes so nice.

Douches can also be used to stem heavy menstruation and to help relieve pain.

Menstrual Disorder Douche

1 tbsp lady's mantle	1 tbsp horsetail
1 tbsp yarrow	½ litre (1 pint) water

Make an infusion. Strain and add six tablespoons to your douche bag. Make up a decoction with one tablespoon of finely chopped angelica root and one tablespoon of rosemary to a litre ($1\frac{3}{4}$ pints) of water and drink three cups of this daily. Warm angelica tea sweetened with a little honey tastes nicer than the cold tea. It will help to make difficult menstruation easier. Do not overdo it. Three cups a day should be sufficient.

I found using this combination of the douche and the tea most helpful for the first few months after I had had a coil fitted, which induced much heavier menstruation than usual.

Chapter 6
The Extremities

Hands

If you despair of your hands you could try the Victorian approach and wear gloves all the time, but the refined ladies who did so then did not have to change nappies, mend cars or dig the garden. Nor did they have to contend with detergents. Hands can never be too clean but they can be harshly cleaned too often and detergents dry out and damage the skin. Wearing rubber gloves while washing up is one solution. Or, better still, wearing a liberal application of hand cream, a pair of cotton gloves and then rubber gloves on top of that. It's effective but it makes me feel like Minnie Mouse and turns me into the world's most adept crockery smasher. The Spanish describe the feeling perfectly: 'a cat with gloves on does not catch any mice'. Instead, I keep a big pot of my own special hand treatment by the sink and after washing up and running my hands in cool running water I dry them well and apply a generous dollop. I always wear cotton gloves for gardening, applying a bit of hand cream first, but if I am embroiled in a really long session I make sure I take them off every hour or so and rinse my hands in cool running water. Working hands perspire in gloves and the acids from trapped perspiration do not do nails any good.

Glove Treatments

I prefer using the glove treatment when I am sleeping alone. Gloves oozing with oatmeal, ground nuts and herbs could be grounds for divorce! But while a glove treatment is by far the most softening and conditioning form of hand care do not use it if you suffer from arthritis or rheumatism in your hands.

First, buy yourself a pair of cheap cotton gloves two sizes too large for you, together with a pair of those very thin plastic disposable gloves one size larger than the cotton ones. These go over the cotton gloves and stop the paste inside oozing out all over the sheets.

Elizabethan ladies used to use kid gloves, which are ideal because they are more or less waterproof, but these seem rather too expensive to be soiled with pomades and masks. The Victorians were particularly keen on glove treatments and advocated the use of oatmeal or pulverized nuts mixed with honey and egg yolks to form a gluey pomade.

Glove Treatment with Nuts

2 heaped tbsp hazelnuts or almonds

1 tbsp clear honey

1 beaten egg yolk

Roast the hazelnuts lightly, then skin and pulverize them or, if using almonds, immerse them in boiling hot water to loosen the skins, skin and pulverize them. Stir in the honey and the egg yolk so the whole mixture forms a squidgey paste. Spread it thickly all over the hands and try, if you can, to get someone to help you into your second glove.

Stain removing Glove Treatment

30 g (1 oz) sorrel leaves

3 heaped tbsp pulverized skinned almonds

1 tbsp orange flower water

6 drops simple tincture of benzoin

milk

Pound the sorrel leaves to a paste and pulverize the skinned almonds. Add the simple tincture of benzoin, the orange flower water and enough milk to form the whole into a paste.

Massage it well into the hands. Apply the gloves and leave on all night.

For Chapped Hands

2 whole houseleeks

4 lady's mantle leaves

1 tbsp honey

1 tsp almond oil

oatmeal

First, express the juice from the houseleeks by liquidizing, then straining them. Save the juice and keep on one side. Shred the lady's mantle finely, then pound it with a pestle and mortar. Gently warm the almond oil and honey together until the honey is dissolved in the oil. Beat in the pulverized lady's mantle, then add the houseleek juice and enough finely ground oatmeal to form a paste. Spread this thickly on to the hands. Apply the gloves and wear all night. This mixture can be stored in a sterilized jar and will keep for a week or two.

Herbal Stain Remover

'To take stains out of ones hands presently.
You may do this with the juice of Sorrell washing the stained place therein.'

Sir Hugh Platt, *Delightes for Ladies*, 1594

Tobacco had only just been introduced to Elizabethan England so presumably nicotine stain removal was not in great demand. Nicotine on the fingers can be removed over a period of time with persistent applications of raw potato juice or lemon juice, or by rubbing the stain vigorously with the inside of any citrus peel. If you want to be really radical you can use equal proportions of hydrogen peroxide and witchhazel and, of course, there is always sorrel juice, which works well but much more gently.

To Soften Hard Skin

Massage a teaspoon of coarse sea salt mixed with a teaspoon of almond oil vigorously into the hardened areas. Do not neglect horny elbows and knees. Then hop into a bath to which you have added more oil and keep the massaged areas immersed in the water for at least ten minutes. Rub away the hard skin with a pumice stone and be lavish with the body lotion.

Of course, you can treat other parts of your body to a mask, the only difficulty being it is harder to keep the mask on, say, your legs than it is on your face.

Mask for Horny Skin

30 g (1 oz) soapwort	half an avocado
basin of water	bran
1 slice of pineapple or pawpaw	4 marshmallow leaves

Finely shred and then pound the marshmallow leaves. Dice the flesh of the fruit. Add this to the marshmallow and pound to a pulp. Add enough bran to make the whole mixture adhere. Soak the horny area for fifteen minutes in a bowl of warm water in which 30 g (1 oz) soapwort has been infused. Dry the skin; spread on the mask in a thick layer. Leave on for twenty minutes then wash off. *Never* try to pare off horny skin with a razor blade.

Horsetail and Meadowsweet Hand Cream

Horsetail is the finest remedy I know for red puffy hands and cracked peeling nails. It is bursting with silicon, which can be directly assimilated by the body, and helps to strengthen the nails and the cuticles. As it is full of calcium it also helps to get rid of the white spots on the fingernails which are signs of decalcification. My own special hand treatment contains both horsetail and meadowsweet which is also rich in calcium. There is still some debate about whether calcium actually does

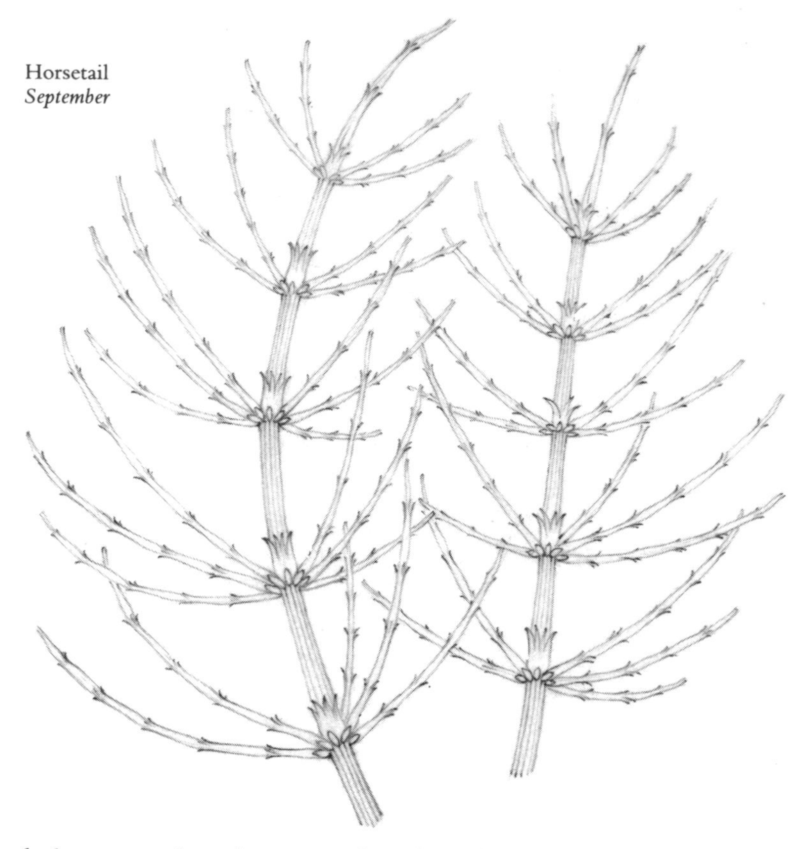
Horsetail
September

help strengthen bones and nails. I believe it does and have listed all the herbs rich in calcium in Chapter 2. They can be taken daily internally in decoctions and infusions to strengthen the nails and used externally as hand and foot soaks. Drink three cups daily and you will see a noticeable improvement in a fortnight and an excellent one in six weeks.

60 g (2 oz) horsetail

60 g (2 oz) meadowsweet

4 cups water

40 ml (1½ fl oz) almond oil

30 g (1 oz) beeswax

20 ml (¾ fl oz or 4 tsp) wheatgerm oil

1½ tbsp clear honey

5 drops essential oil of chamomile

Gently simmer the herbs in the water in a covered enamel saucepan for half an hour. Leave covered and allow to cool. Strain through a coffee filter paper. Melt the almond oil and the beeswax together in a double boiler. Add the honey and stir this into the mixture. Add the strained herbal decoction and the wheatgerm oil and beat thoroughly. Finally, beat in the essential oil and stir slowly until the cream is cool. Use this superbly soothing hand cream often in small quantities, paying special attention to the cuticles.

Liver Spots

Liver spots are a problem I'm often asked about. They are large brown spots which usually appear on the back of hands and seem to be the result of age and lack of vitamins E, C and B_2. The age you can't do anything about, but you can rub wheatgerm oil into the spots nightly and step up your intake of vitamin C and the B complex vitamins. The freckle removers mentioned in Chapter 7 may also help as will Sir Hugh Platt's recommendation:

To take away spots and freckles from the face or hands
'Take sappe that issueth out of a Birch tree in great abundance, being opened, in March or April, with a receiver of glasse set under the boring there to receive the same, doth perform the same most excellently, and maketh the skin very clear.'

Delightes for Ladies, 1594

For instructions on how to bleed a birch tree, see p. 71.

Exercise for the Hands

Hands, more than any other part of the body, can get overused and feel cramped. (As the first draft of this book was written in longhand I speak with the voice of authority!) Revitalize your hands by trying to bring all the fingertips on one hand simultaneously to the points where the finger joints meet the upper pads of the palm. Stretch your fingers out in full extension.

Hold for a few seconds. Relax. Let the fingers dangle for a moment. Repeat several times. Repeat with the other hand.

Warts

There are all sorts of extraordinary folk remedies for removing warts. A traditional cure dating back to well before the fourteenth century suggests:

'Put three drops of blood from a wart into an Elder leaf, and bury it in the earth repeating this charm –
Three drops of blood put in thee
Deare leafe of goode Eldern tree,
And bury thee; thou'll rot away,
Then my warts will fast decay!'

Cures which work for nearly all wart sufferers are double-strength infusions of any of the following herbs: bluebell flowers, ivy leaves, the juice squeezed from the stem of greater celandine and the sap extracted from marigold leaves.

To take warts away
'To take green leaves of Marigold, and beat them to mash in a Mortar, so that upon pressing it the Juice be apt to come out. With this Juice – mash rub your warts well three or four times a day.'
Ram's Little Dodeon, 1606

Gerard recommended a decoction of rampion root. Rampion was a popular pot herb in Elizabethan times: the roots, which have the sweetish taste of parsnip, were boiled and served with a sauce. You can grow your own rampion from seeds obtained from a herb nursery. It likes a moist sandy soil.

Whichever herb you decide upon, rub a strong infusion or decoction on to the wart daily. A piece of lint soaked in the infusion should be applied over the wart and secured with a bandage. The dressing should be changed twice daily. Do not apply a dressing if using greater celandine. Take care to rub this only on the wart. If you spread it on the surrounding

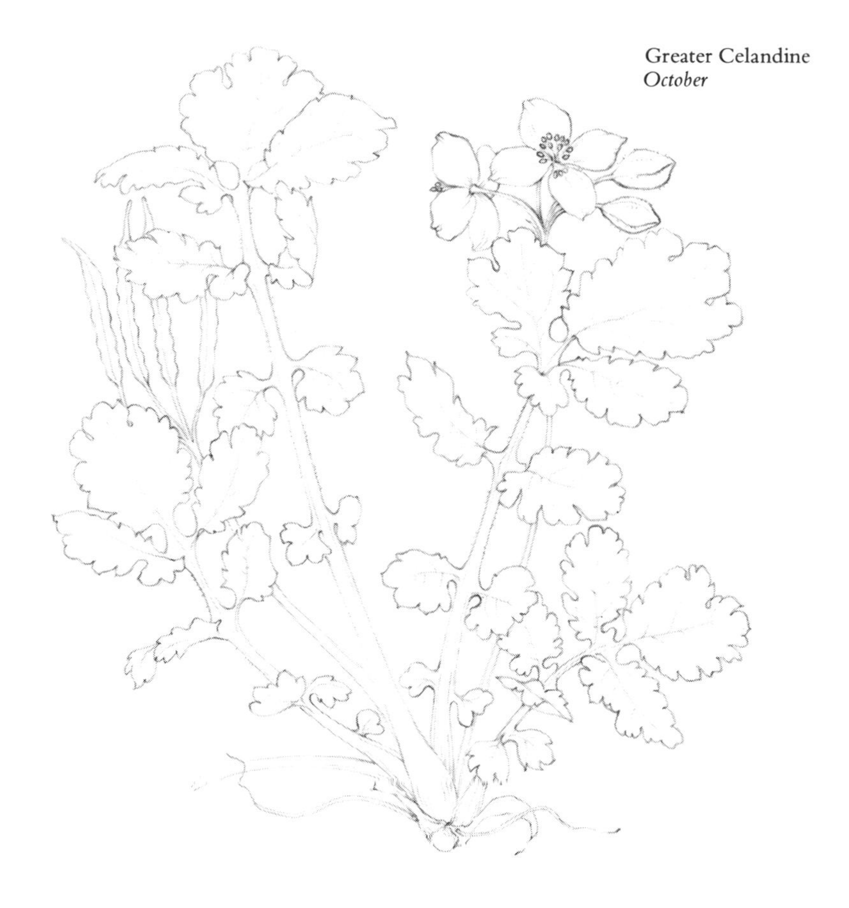
Greater Celandine
October

skin it will cause it to crack and flake. In a week or two the wart will soften and eventually disappear.

Chilblains

The Romans, transported from the delights of sunny Italy to the rigours of a winter manning Hadrian's Wall, used to stimulate their frozen limbs by flogging themselves with nettles. A somewhat radical solution to chilblains. Here are a few solutions which are far less radical and absolutely painless, even if some of them are a bit inconvenient.

To Soothe Chilblains

Cut a leaf of houseleek lengthways and rub the exposed juicy flesh over the chilblains twice daily.

To Prevent Chilblains

Lightly crush some strawberries and bandage them to the area where you usually get chilblains. Keep on overnight, covering the bandages with plastic if necessary to prevent strawberry juice staining the sheets. Keep this treatment up for a week and it will prevent the onset of chilblains in the winter. This treatment can be carried out at any time in the summer when strawberries are plentiful.

Broken Chilblains

Soak broken chilblains in a warm infusion of marigold flowers nightly, then cover with a lukewarm poultice of the strained-out petals, kept in place with a bandage. Put on a pair of thick socks if the chilblains are on your feet, as the poultice tends to ooze through the bandages. Lumber into bed. Throw away the poultice in the morning and repeat the marigold soak. This relieves the agony of broken chilblains very quickly and accelerates their healing.

Nails

Nail care is obviously an integral part of hand care. The nail plate from which your nail grows is several millimetres below the base of the nail and it takes about nine months for a new nail to grow, though even this process slows down as you grow older. Nails indicate your state of health just as clearly as the condition of your skin, eyes and hair. Pale nails with vertical ridges indicate anaemia or extreme dryness from using too many detergents. Blue nails point to inefficient circulation or not enough oxygen. If your nails are thin and constantly breaking this may indicate inadequate vitamins, minerals and protein, as well as insufficient nail care and perhaps the use of metal nail manicure sets which are not good for encouraging strong healthy nails.

Diet for Strengthening Nails

Plenty of horsetail tea, calcium, gelatine and vitamin B complex. Vitamin D cures vertical ridges, folic acid and vitamin C cures hangnails and split nails. The former, which are cracks in the skin along the sides of the nails, can be particularly painful. Drink diluted cider vinegar to strengthen nails and paint them with two coats of fresh lemon juice daily to strengthen them externally. Always remember to put on a pair of cotton-lined gloves before tackling jobs that involve the use of detergents. Hangnails should be treated with lavish applications of the horsetail and iris hand cream and the tip of dry skin which develops should be cut off carefully rather than pulled, to prevent damage of the surrounding skin.

Nail Care

This includes toenails, which may be harder to reach, but then, considerately, they grow a little more slowly than fingernails. Once a week soak your hands and feet in a warm decoction of horsetail and soapwort. Then take an orange stick with a rubber pad on the end and gently push back the cuticles. If you cannot get hold of a hoof stick use Q-tips or an orange stick with the tip wrapped in sterile cotton. Clean under the nails with a natural bristle brush. If you are wearing nail polish remove it with acetone mixed with a few drops of glycerine or castor oil. Acetone is very drying, so these additions will help, but be meticulous about removing every trace of acetone from the corners of the nails – to be doubly sure soak the nails again. Rinse the hands in cool water and dry. File the nails with an emeryboard, following the natural curve of the nail. Never use a metal file, which only tears at the edges of the nails. Do not cut the cuticles with one of those nail-clipping gadgets or with

Alkanet Leaves and Flower
October

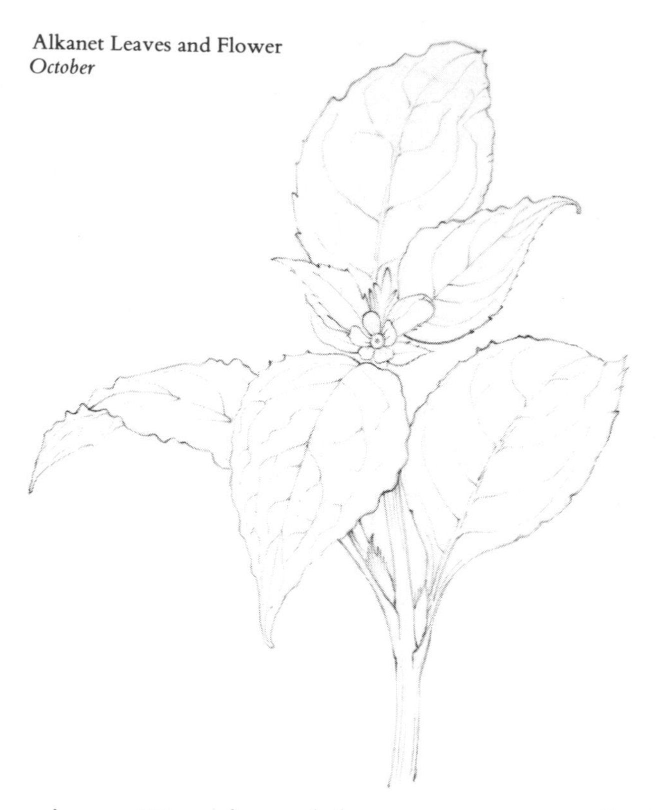

scissors. Wrongly used they can cause a lot of pain and damage.

Massage the nail with a cuticle cream to bring the blood up to the surface of the finger and help the matrix from which the nail grows. If you want to stimulate the circulation and strengthen the nails even more buff them with a chamois leather pad.

Iris and Horsetail Cuticle Cream

30 g (1 oz) horsetail

30 g (1 oz) iris (flowers)

1 cup water

4 tbsp anhydrous lanolin

1 tsp powdered lecithin

1 tsp glycerine

5 drops essential oil of roses

Simmer the horsetail, iris flowers and water in a covered enamel double boiler for an hour (the use of a double boiler will prevent the fragile iris petals catching and burning). Strain out the decoction through coffee filter paper and set aside. Melt the lanolin and lecithin together in a double boiler, beat in the glycerine and slowly add the herbal decoction, beating hard. Allow the cream to cool to blood heat and stir in the essential oil.

Colouring Nails

Nails can be coloured naturally by using henna paste, which should be painted on the nails and left for ten minutes to an hour depending on how deep you want the colour to be. They can also be coloured with alkanet, from which a deep red dye can be extracted by macerating the root in oil. Alkanet is most often found growing in hedgerows. It looks very similar to borage – it even has the same soft downy texture – but it can be differentiated by the flowers, which are rounded at the end instead of star-shaped. The bright azure blue flowers, unlike borage flowers, all grow on the same side of the terminal spike. The root, which is the part you will want to use, is very large – quite out of proportion to the rest of the plant. There is an illustration of alkanet opposite and one of borage on plate 4 so you can compare the two herbs.

Alkanet Colouring

30 g (1 oz) alkanet root, finely chopped

60 ml (2 fl oz) almond oil

15 g (½ oz) hydrous lanolin

essential oil of your choice (optional)

Pound the alkanet root to a paste. Add the oil and scrape the mixture into a jar. Seal tightly and macerate for a fortnight. Strain through coffee filter paper. Melt the lanolin in a double boiler. Beat in the oil and add a few drops of any essential oil of your choice at this point, if your want the colouring to smell nice. My own favourites are chamomile or neroli. Rub the colouring carefully into the nails trying not to let it overlap on the cuticles. If it does, clean the cuticles quickly with a Q-tip dipped in soapy water to prevent them becoming stained red. The longer you leave the colour on, the deeper red it will become. Rinse your hands, then gild the lily by buffing your nails. Like henna, the colour will last for weeks. It will not wash off but it will eventually wear off and, of course, grow out as your nails grow. It tends to wear off fairly evenly.

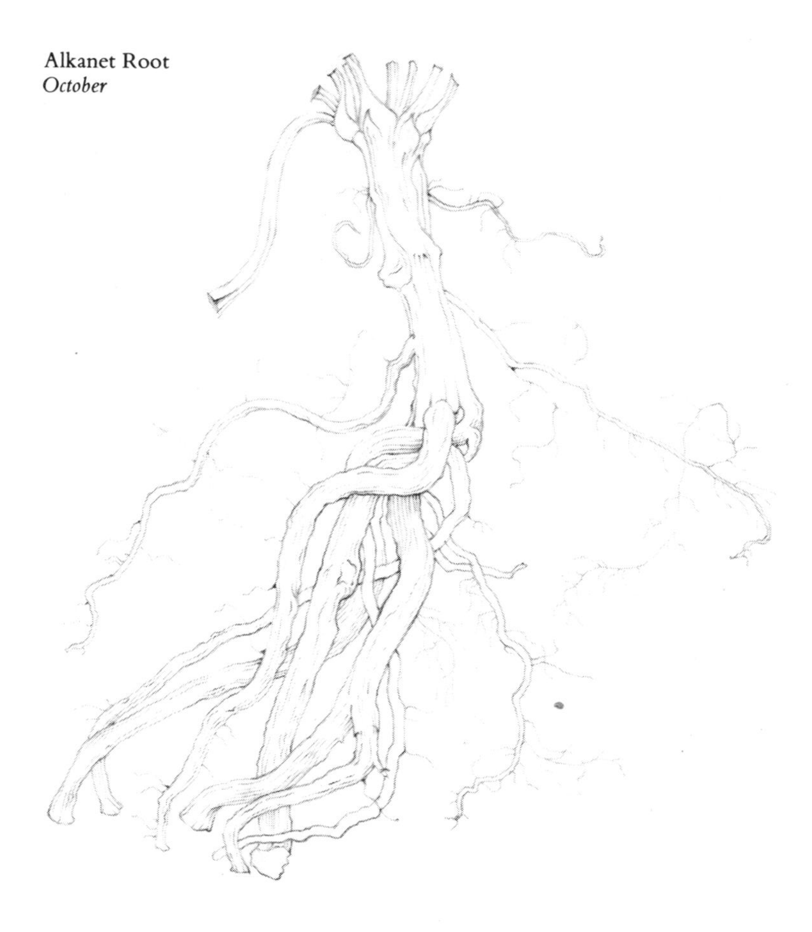

Alkanet Root
October

Feet

Have you noticed how ugly most people's feet are? It is through neglect rather than the way mother made them. Feet are the hardest working part of your body. They contain almost a quarter of all the bones in the body and da Vinci quite rightly pronounced them the 'greatest engineering device in the world'.

The first and most important rule is to wear shoes that fit. Corns and callouses are caused by pressure from badly fitted shoes.

Ivy Corn Remover

Macerate 30 g (1 oz) of ivy leaves in enough cider vinegar to barely cover in a sealed jar. Leave to stand for a fortnight topping up with vinegar from time to time if necessary. Fork out one of the leaves and bind it on to the corn with a piece of linament and a bandage. Change the leaf and the dressing twice daily and gradually the corn will become soft enough to lift out. Lavish lots of marigold moisturizer, (p. 182) on your feet until the scar heals and then switch to a daily massage with the horsetail and meadowsweet hand cream, (p. 149).

Refreshing Foot Herbs

There is no better way to refresh tired feet than with a foot bath. Add any of the herbs below to freshly boiled water and then allow the water to cool to blood heat. Immerse your feet in the water. Wriggle your toes, which will help ease aching arches, then relax.

elderberries

ferns

mugwort

nettles

peppermint

pine needles

rosemary

sage

yarrow

Alternatively, you can make up a decoction of mustard seed (2 heaped tablespoons to 3 litres ($5\frac{1}{4}$ pints) of water) or, if you really want to dance the light fantastic all night, massage your feet with a teaspoon of wheatgerm oil in which you have mixed half a teaspoon of lavender oil. Then immerse them in one of the foot baths above. Also very invigorating is 1 tablespoon of avocado oil, 1 tablespoon coarse sea salt and 15 drops of marigold or rosemary oil rubbed firmly and vigorously into the feet before soaking in a foot bath.

Foot Massage

A foot massage is my idea of heaven and is the surest way of getting not just your feet but your whole body to relax. A massage will also improve the circulation and soothe swollen feet. Try getting someone who loves you to do it for you. If you have to go it alone start kneading the sole of one foot with your bunched fist. Now hold the foot between both hands, first giving a circular thumb massage all over the top, then to the bottom of the foot. Rub the ankle in a wide circular motion with your fingertips. Run your thumb firmly along each tendon on top of the foot, working upwards towards the ankle and at the same time squeezing the foot with a hard pumping action between your hands. Now massage each toe individually with a spiralling movement. The whole thing is easier if you first anoint your feet with a herbal oil or do it in soapy bath water. The first time you try this you will understand why it is easier to let someone else give you the massage. All that stretching to reach and hold the feet is quite a strain, especially if you are blessed with long legs. You can also try this massage using a vibrator, which is easier than using your own fingers, does an adequate job (though not as effective as a hand massage) but is not recommended for those who have ticklish feet.

William Coles in *The Art of Simpling* observed 'if a Footman take Mugwort and put into his shoes in the Morning, he may go forty Miles before Noon and not be weary'. Ferns and elderberry leaves stuffed into the shoes also relieve fatigue. The country people used to stuff their shoes with greater mullein leaves to cushion their feet against rough roads.

Soothing Foot Baths

These can be concocted using an infusion of geranium leaves, lady's mantle, comfrey, marshmallows and houseleek. Add a dash of cider vinegar to the water as well. After soaking the feet treat them to a generous rub with any of the creams you would use for your hands. Cold feet can be warmed by a dash of cayenne pepper diluted with a little talc sprinkled into the socks or, better still, by moving both feet from hot to cold foot baths, ending with a cold bath and a vigorous rub with a rough towel. This really gets the circulation moving and so warms your feet, though the first dip in the cold basin requires a bit of courage.

Athlete's Foot

This is a fungal ringworm infection which makes the feet feel itchy, unusually moist and unpleasantly smelly. The pH of the foot changes from its normal acid balance to an alkaline one. The way to correct this is to change the pH back to acid by using cider vinegar foot baths three times daily. I have come across recommendations to piss between the toes, which is where the worst of the infection usually is. This makes sense as far as the acid argument is concerned, but women will obviously find it difficult to accomplish.

People with athlete's foot should use soapwort not soap to wash the feet, which should always be kept scrupulously clean and absolutely dry. The feet should be allowed as much air and sun as possible but be considerate about walking around with bare feet in public places: athlete's foot is highly infectious.

Herbal Bath for Athlete's Foot

30 g (1 oz) red clover

30 g (1 oz) sage

30 g (1 oz) marigolds

30 g (1 oz) agrimony

3 litres (5¼ pints) water

2 tbsp cider vinegar

Make a decoction of the herbs by simmering them in the water for twenty minutes. Strain. Allow to cool and add the cider vinegar just before immersing your feet. Save the strained herbs to use as a poultice, spreading them thickly between the toes. An empty basin placed beneath your feet during this operation will catch the bits that drop off. Relax. Watch your favourite television programme – something that lasts about half an hour is the right duration. Then rinse your feet and dry meticulously. Powder them with arrowroot.

Excessive Perspiration of the Feet

If you try to suppress this it will only lead to all sorts of other damage like skin eruptions as the result of toxins being trapped inside the body. Perspiration can be minimized by drinking diuretic teas like lady's mantle, couchgrass, dandelion, thyme, fennel seed, parsley and pennyroyal. Foot baths containing the same herbs can also be used. Sprinkling the feet with neat witchhazel and making sure you spread your toes so that the skin between them is well doused also helps. Wait a few seconds, towel away any excess moisture that has not evaporated and then apply lots of corn starch. Never wear heavy socks, especially those made from synthetic fibres: they prime feet for sweating. Go around barefoot or in leather sandals as much as possible.

Foot Deodorants

All the advice offered for perspiring feet applies. Try a double-strength infusion of lovage or cleavers or a decoction of white willow bark in a foot bath daily. These will act as natural deodorants.

Exercises for the Feet

Picking up marbles with your toes strengthens your feet and your arches. If you have long since lost all your marbles try using pencils or paintbrushes instead. Swim as much as you can. Walk barefoot on flat surfaces as often as possible. Firm sandy beaches are ideal for this as well as being enjoyable. Lying with your feet propped up higher than your head for half an hour daily helps to take the pressure off thread veins and relieves aching legs.

Chapter 7
Problems

Wrinkles

While it's true that the only way to rejuvenate a wrinkled face is by cosmetic surgery – a somewhat radical and expensive step – there are a few preventive measures you can take to stave off the evil day.

Anti-wrinkle measures

Avoid long exposure to the sun. As well as increasing the possibility of skin cancer the sun's searing rays attack the collagen fibres which support the skin and give it its elasticity. Once they collapse, wrinkles will set in for life, unless they are artificially removed with the surgeon's knife.

There is a school of thought which suggests that crow's feet become more deeply etched if you smoke. Quite why this should be so has never been clear to me except that presumably heavy smokers squint more than non-smokers do in order to protect their eyes from the smoke. The warnings emblazoned on cigarette packets are enough to remind you that smoking is dangerously unhealthy so I won't preach to confirmed addicts. If you must pollute your body, just bear in mind the physiological fact that the skin around the eyes is drier than that on the rest of the face, so wrinkles will appear here more quickly than in other areas. Treat the eye area to plenty of water and lavish amounts of light moisturizer.

The right amount of sleep produces a less lined complexion. If you don't believe this go to a few all-night parties and then peer closely at your skin. Anxiety, tension and stress are also all sure-fire ageing factors (see Chapter 8).

The skin needs moisture to look and stay young. Neglect the moisturizing process and you will accelerate the appearance of wrinkles. A good anti-wrinkle cream will contain the right balance of oils to lubricate the skin and water to moisturize it.

Nourish yourself internally and you will fend off the wrinkles externally. Eat a good helping of protein daily, otherwise your body will have to resort to using its own stored protein and, as the muscles begin to give way, wrinkles will set in. Make sure you are getting all the necessary vitamins (you should be if you are following a balanced diet) and take in some extra vitamin B complex, especially B_2, riboflavin, found in liver and milk.

The debate as to whether facial exercise helps still rages. In theory it should because the enlargement of a mass of muscle means you stretch the skin and smooth it out. On the other hand you have to indulge in a lot of gymnastics to increase a bicep even slightly, which is discouraging as far as the face is concerned. Imagine the amount of effort required to remove etched forehead wrinkles. It is probably more important to learn to relax your facial muscles, thus smoothing out the wrinkles which are symptomatic of tension than to exercise them. But it is hard to relax them without consciously recognizing what the opposite feeling is like. So go ahead and scream silently, yawn, pout, grin, sneer, whistle, puff up your cheeks, wrinkle your nose, open your eyes so wide that they feel as if they are popping out. Now relax your facial muscles. Let all the tension flow out of you and focus your eyes and concentrate your internal gaze on the spot between your eyebrows. Luxuriate in the warm place you have just created for yourself. Next time you frown or squint remember how much nicer it feels to have a relaxed face. Also bear in mind that when you frown you use forty-four face muscles, but when you smile you use only fourteen.

There are herbs which not only soften and lubricate the skin, but which are believed to help in cell regeneration:

Anti-wrinkle Herbs

comfrey

elderflowers

fennel

honeysuckle flowers

houseleek

lady's mantle

lime blossom

marshmallow

narcissus roots
(a favourite Roman anti-wrinkle herb)

white lily root
(a popular Victorian anti-wrinkle herb)

Anti-wrinkle Cream

30 g (1 oz) beeswax

15 g ($\frac{1}{2}$ oz) clear honey

90 ml (3 fl oz) avocado oil

30 ml (1 fl oz) wheatgerm oil

30 ml (1 fl oz) of an infusion or decoction of any one of the anti-wrinkle herbs, using 30 g (1 oz) of the herb to 2 cups of water

6 drops tincture of myrrh

3 drops essential oil of honeysuckle

Follow the Basic Cream Directions on p. 57, first melting the honey with the beeswax.

This cream can also be rubbed under the eyes providing you are not allergic to the beeswax or myrrh in it. If you are, substitute anhydrous lanolin for the beeswax and omit the myrrh. Another excellent anti-wrinkle cream is the mayonnaise skin food described on p. 80.

Anti-wrinkle Wash

Prepare a strong infusion of poppy flowers using 60 g (2 oz) flowers to a litre (1¾ pints) of water. Spray this liberally on to your face using a plant mister before applying the anti-wrinkle cream.

The French recommend stretching the wrinkled area with two fingers and making sure it stays smooth and taut by sticking a strip of sellotape over the area. I find elastoplast on less delicate areas of the body excruciating enough to remove; sellotape around the eyes strikes me as masochism.

Acne

Acne is the result of uncontrolled blackheads and pimples exploding into pussy spots and running riot because of increased hormone production which over-stimulates the sebaceous glands. It is normally a problem which occurs in adolescence, when there is a sudden increase of both female and male hormone production, but acne is not uncommon in adults.

Acne Activators

Tension plays havoc with the hormonal balance in the body, increasing the two things acne sufferers could do without: oily secretions and perspiration.

Too much iodine in the system stimulates acne. Iodine is found in spices, shellfish and, of course, in iodized salt.

Chocolate, nuts, white sugar and all other stodgy and fatty foods give acne a helping hand.

An Anti-acne Way of Life

A way of life I'm afraid it has to be because this problem will not clear up overnight. But the following steps, if faithfully adhered to, will help reduce and finally clear up the acne altogether.

Try and become a more relaxed person. Easier said than done, I know, if you are nervously inclined. The suggestions in Chapter 8 will help.

Avoid all iodized, fatty, sugar foods and chocolates. Instead, make sure you incorporate two tablespoons of any vegetable oil into your diet daily; also niacin and vitamins C and A. Use toasted and ground sesame seeds (which are full of niacin) to replace salt. They taste slightly spicy and very pleasant. A pepper mill makes a very satisfactory grinder.

Keep your skin sparkling clean and at all costs avoid the temptation of picking at pussy spots. If you have oozing pustular acne avoid facial steams. Use a daily mask instead and wait until the spots have healed over before steaming. Use a soapwort wash in preference to ordinary soap.

A little gentle sunbathing helps.

Healing Herbs for Acne

burdock

comfrey

fresh violet leaves

horsetail

inner bark of dried elm

inner bark of dried white willow

lavender

leaves and flowers of wild pansy

soapwort

sorrel

A combination of any of the herbs above can be used in a facial steam. The elm and white willow barks will need to be made up as a decoction and then can be added to an infusion of the other herbs. You can strain off the water after a facial steam and use this to pat on to the acne during the course of the day. All these herbs will also help taken internally as a tea three times daily. I have achieved some notable successes by prescribing burdock tea. Lavender tea is particularly useful here, as it gradually helps to normalize the secretions from the sebaceous glands. You can make a stronger form of lavender tea using the stalks and flowers in a home-made still. Do not use commercial lavender water because the alcohol in it will prove agonizing on tender broken skins.

Violet Leaf Mask

Take a large handful of violet leaves. Pound them to a pulp and apply as a mask. Violets have remarkable antiseptic properties and are excellent for keeping the skin scrupulously clean.

Charcoal Mask

Grill three pieces of wholemeal bread until they are burnt to a cinder. Mix with a tablespoon of clear honey and spread this thickly on the face.

Onion and White Willow Poultice

Make a double-strength decoction of white willow bark using 30 g (1 oz) of bark to half a litre (¾ pint) of water. Chop up one large onion and simmer it in four tablespoons of the decoction until it is reduced to a pulp. Make the pulp into a poultice (see Chapter 1) and apply this while it is still warm to the acne. Wash off with any left-over decoction. The salicylic acid in the bark and the sulphur in the onion are both very helpful acne remedies.

All the above masks can be used daily, but do not expect miracles in a week. A couple of months of persistent treatment will produce dividends. Remember to treat yourself internally as well with daily herbal teas: a mixture of burdock, inner bark of elm, lavender and marigolds is particularly helpful.

Eczema

Eczema is a term which does not embrace a single skin disease but a whole group of skin eruptions characterized by very dry scaly skin which usually occurs in all the most awkward places – the face, elbows, wrists, backs of hands and behind the knees. Sometimes it appears as weeping sores.

An Anti-eczema Way of Life

Like acne, eczema can be aggravated by tension, so rule one for acne should be followed.

Dry weather, strong soaps and too many showers and baths all make the problem worse. Avoid direct exposure to the sun and wear light cotton clothes as much as you can. They help the skin breathe and do not irritate like wool does. When you take a bath add eczema-healing herbs wrapped in a square of muslin. Wash with handfuls of finely ground oatmeal instead of soap. Keep the skin as moisturized as possible.

Step up the vitamin B content in your diet, particularly pyridoxine, B_6, and B_{12}. Take at least two tablespoons a day of soy, safflower, corn, sunflower or avocado oil.

Above all, try not to scratch, which only makes the condition much worse.

Itchy Eczema

When the itching gets unbearable, apply a poultice of finely grated fresh carrot or grate one tablespoon of fresh horseradish. Mix either of these into a small tub of plain yoghurt. Leave this to macerate for an hour then strain out the carrot or horseradish. Apply this as a paste to the itchy bits. Alternatively, spread a thin layer of live plain yoghurt on to the skin. Leave it on for as long as you can, then rinse off gently with tepid water. Freshly squeezed lemon juice, diluted 1:3 with purified water, also soothes itching eczema. Dab it on liberally as often as required.

Potato Mask

Some people find a finely grated raw potato applied as a mask helps. But be careful; I have known people who are allergic to raw potato. Try a patch test first.

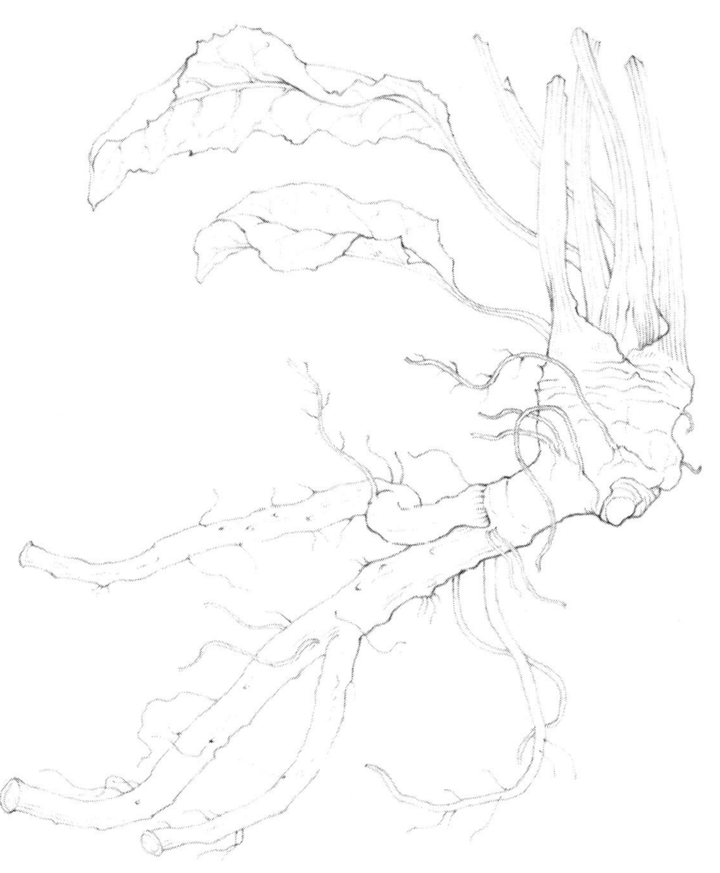

Horseradish
August

Soothing Juice for Eczema

Cut a houseleek leaf through lengthways, separating the top surface of the leaf from the bottom surface so that a large expanse of juicy flesh is exposed (an illustration of the correct way to cut a houseleek leaf is included on Plate 8). Rub this on the eczema.

Eczema-relieving Herbs

- bay leaves
- bilberry leaves
- cabbage
- celandine (see warning on p. 152)
- chamomile
- cleavers
- comfrey
- daisy
- dandelion
- horseradish root
- houseleek
- lime flowers
- marshmallow
- plantain
- sage
- silver birch bark
- strawberry leaves
- walnut leaves
- watercress

Bruise a combination of any of these herbs slightly with a pestle and mortar, and tie them up in a large muslin square to which you have added a handful of oatmeal. You can use the bath bag to wash your skin lightly once it has been immersed in your bath water for a good ten minutes.

Eczema Moisturizer

30 g (1 oz) comfrey

30 g (1 oz) chamomile

30 g (1 oz) watercress

30 g (1 oz) celery seeds (powdered)

90 ml (3 fl oz) wheatgerm oil

90 ml (3 fl oz) almond oil

30 ml (1 fl oz) linseed oil

Pound up the comfrey, chamomile and watercress to a paste with a pestle and mortar. Stir in the powdered celery seeds. Add the mixture to a jar containing the three oils and mash them well into the oil. Seal tightly. Macerate for two weeks. Strain out the herbs through coffee filter paper. Use the resulting thick green oil sparingly to moisturize your skin or add a teaspoon of it to your bath water. If you cannot buy refined linseed oil, increase the quantity of almond oil appropriately.

Psoriasis

Psoriasis is the result of the epidermis producing skin at nearly ten times the normal rate so that it bunches up into ridges and scales and continually flakes off. You will have gathered from the description that it is a miserably debilitating disease which, not surprisingly, causes the sufferer great distress. There is still some debate as to whether diet can actually help, but it certainly would not do any harm to apply the same dietary principles used for eczema to this disease. In addition, psoriasis sufferers should drink decoctions of the inner bark of elm or infusions of birch leaves three times daily. The skin needs to be kept as soft and as supple as possible, which can be done by using lanolin mixed with a little wheatgerm oil and infusions or decoctions of the following herbs:

Psoriasis-relieving Herbs

birch leaves

chamomile

comfrey

houseleek

inner bark of elm or white willow

marshmallow

motherwort

Bruise all the herbs first with a pestle and mortar. These can be used in the bath by selecting a combination of the herbs and tying up a good handful in a muslin square. Place the muslin bag on the worst affected areas, but do not rub the skin with it. After the bath pat, don't rub yourself dry and apply the following salve to the worst affected places:

Psoriasis Salve

30 g (1 oz) comfrey

30 g (1 oz) houseleek

30 g (1 oz) of the soft inner bark of elm

3 cups water

60 g (2 oz) anhydrous lanolin

30 ml (1 fl oz) wheatgerm oil

Chop up the comfrey and houseleek as finely as possible and break up the bark into tiny bits. Simmer in three cups of water in a tightly covered enamel saucepan for half an hour. Allow to cool. Strain through coffee filter paper. Melt the lanolin, beat in the wheatgerm oil and as much of the decoction as you need to form a runny paste. Rub it gently into the affected areas. You will find a little goes a long way and, though it is somewhat messy to use, it is very effective. I have had some startling successes using this salve which really does help to alleviate and control psoriasis.

I do not often recommend things by name but I feel I must recommend Wright's Coal Tar soap and shampoo for psoriasis. Every other soap and shampoo only seems to make the condition worse. It is probably the tar in the soap which helps this particular skin condition and most of the commercial products used to treat psoriasis contain it.

Treat yourself internally by drinking a daily decoction of the inner bark of elm, 15 g (½ oz) to half a litre (1 pint) of water. Sweeten with honey as it tastes somewhat unpleasant. Above all, refuse to simply give in and learn to live with the disease!

Most sufferers can be helped by careful and persistent adherence to these treatments. Too often people abandon them the moment the condition temporarily improves, which is disastrous as the condition will almost certainly flare up again. Continuous treatment is essential. Psoriasis can be controlled; it cannot be cured.

Spots

Start by tackling the spots from the inside out, because that is where they came from in the first place. No one's skin can thrive on a fatty diet with lots of sweet and starchy foods. Drink plenty of water. Eat lots of fresh fruit, vegetables, low-fat live yoghurt and whole grain foods. Exercises (the secret is regularity, not strenuousness) and fresh air improve the circulation, flushing the blood up to the skin, which in turn helps the skin to fight bacteria and heal more quickly.

Continue your all-out preventative assault by keeping the skin scrupulously clean. If you can keep your pores consistently unclogged you are well on the way to a blemish-free complexion – whiteheads occur because skin pores become plugged with sebum. Once the plug oxidizes it turns dark and becomes a blackhead. The sebum keeps being pumped up to the surface of the skin but it still has no exit and enzymes beaver away on the oils splitting them into irritating acids. The blackheads then become an even larger sore red spot. Eventually the follicle walls rupture under the strain of all that oil, acid and bacteria, flooding the surrounding skin with even more inflammation. More white cells are produced in the blood in an attempt to fight back. These create pus and at this stage you are teetering on the brink of acne. This perverted Pilgrim's Progress of the spot should be enough to induce anyone to tackle the problem when it is at its smallest and simplest. Begin with the whitehead and blackhead.

A Skin Care Routine to Remove Whiteheads and Blackheads (follow these steps in sequence)

Wash with any of the previously mentioned scrubs for oily

skins. Rinse with a warm infusion of violet flowers or comfrey.

Use any of the herbal facial steams recommended for oily skins (see p. 63).

Apply a mask made up of the following ingredients:

1 tsp honey

1 tbsp oatmeal

1 egg white

1 tsp wheatgerm

or apply Parkinson's Lupin Mask for Oily Skin (p. 69)

The women of ancient Greece and Rome were particularly fond of using a paste of crushed lupin seeds to remove skin blemishes. Wash the mask off with lots of tepid water.

Rub the spots with a teaspoon of fine sea salt dampened with a teaspoon of the milky juice crushed from dandelion stalks. At this point most of the pores will have emptied themselves of their plugs. Any remaining blackheads can be squeezed out with clean fingers protected with tissues.

Now disinfect and close the pores with any of the following solutions:

basil wine

cider vinegar

double-strength infusion of violets

elderflower water

lemon juice

thyme vinegar

witchhazel

Measure out 100 ml ($3\frac{1}{3}$ fl oz) of any of the above herbs and mix with 30 ml (1 fl oz) of simple tincture of benzoin.

Spots can be dabbed with any of these solutions frequently during the day.

Stubborn Blackhead Remover

Rub wheatgerm oil into the offending blackhead then use a facial steam. Rub in even more wheatgerm oil and apply flannels to the blackheads as hot as you can stand them. This vigorous treatment softens the blackheads making it easier to push them out. The use of wheatgerm oil makes sure the skin heals over quickly.

Depuratives (herbs which purify the system from the inside and help to ensure a clear skin on the outside) should be taken in tea form daily.

Depurative Herbs

betony
borage
burdock
chickweed
couchgrass
dandelion
elder leaves
lovage
plantain
shepherd's purse
summer savory
watercress

Solutions for the Occasional Pimple

Cut a mistletoe berry in half and rub the spot with the juice of the berry.

Dab it with birch milk.

If the problem hits you in the spring rub the milky sap from the stalk of a daisy on the spot.

Rub the sap from a dandelion on to the spot, but use this treatment overnight as it tends to leave a brown smudge on the skin. Don't be alarmed; it is very temporary.

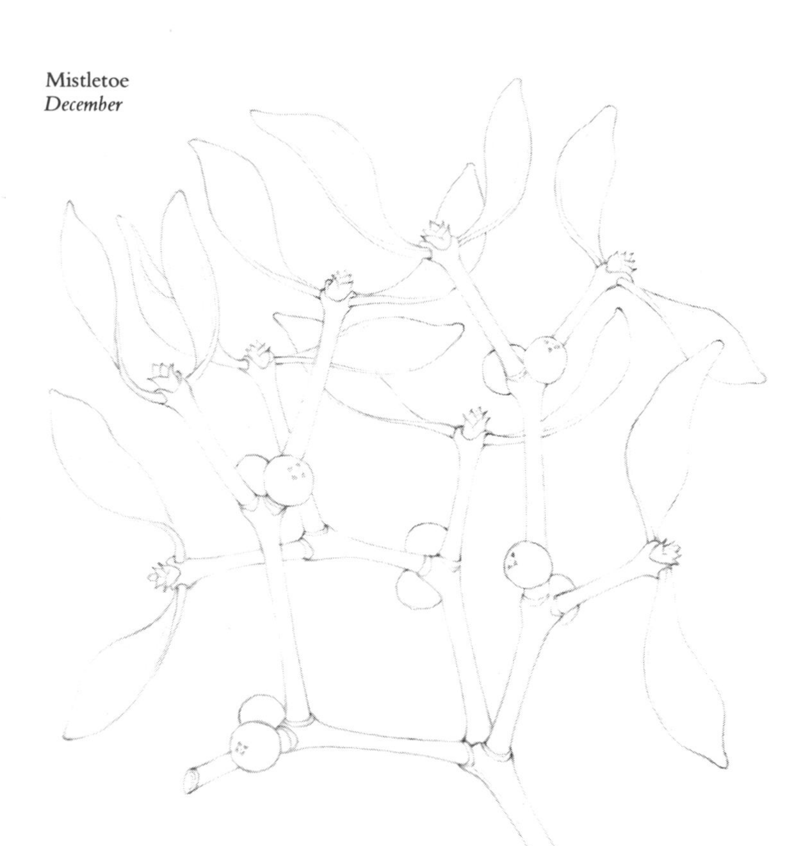
Mistletoe
December

Excessive Redness (Roseola)

This condition, caused by congestion of the capillaries, can be soothed by the daily application of a cold poppy flower poultice. Wild or cultivated poppies may be used (see p. 34 for how to make up a poultice). This should be followed by dabbing the face with lettuce milk.

Lettuce Milk

outer leaves 1 lettuce

water

4 drops simple tincture of benzoin

Use any lettuce for this except an Iceberg or Chinese lettuce. Wash carefully under running water. Put the leaves in an enamel saucepan and barely cover with boiling water. Cover tightly and simmer gently for half an hour. Allow to cool, still covered. Strain the mixture through coffee filter paper and add the tincture of benzoin. Store in a refrigerator.

Wash the face with finely ground oatmeal. Moisturize with the cream recommended for thread veins (see p. 182) and disguise the redness with some of the new green foundation cream specially made to cover birthmarks, but also useful for similar skin conditions. Do not worry; in spite of the colour of the foundation you will not come out green. *Never* use a facial steam and avoid sunbathing. Both only aggravate the problem. A seventeenth-century recipe suggested the following steps:

To cure Excessive Ruddiness of the Face
'It is good overnight to anoint the face with hare's blood and in the morning to wash it with strawberry and cowslip water, the juyce of distil'd lemon, juyce of cowcumbers or to use the seeds of melon or kernels of peaches beaten small.'

Forget the hare's blood. All the other ingredients will certainly help. The lemon juice would have been distilled in an alembick, but in this instance fresh and untreated lemon juice is just as effective.

Freckles

Happily, freckles are not the unfashionable bane they used to be, but if you have so many freckles you can hardly see any skin you may want to help them fade. Stay out of the sun, which only accentuates them, and apply any of the following treatments daily.

Horseradish Yoghurt (see section on eczema, p. 170). This should be dabbed on to the freckles, allowed to dry, then washed off with warm water. Milk may be used in this recipe as an alternative to the yoghurt recommended for eczema.

Rosehip and Cucumber Mask

2 tbsp dried rosehips

2 tsp cucumber juice

Pound the rosehips to a powder. Mix to a paste with the cucumber juice and apply this mask to the freckles for fifteen minutes.

Marie Antoinette was particularly fond of a buttermilk compress to remove freckles. For instructions on how to prepare a compress see p. 32. Apply the compress cold in this instance.

Victorian beauties used three parts of fresh lemon juice mixed with one part rum to dab on their freckles.

Try washes from strawberry leaves and ivy leaves boiled in just enough wine to cover, or elder leaves. The last suggestion comes from the following recipe:

To Take Away Freckles and Morphew
'Distil Elder Leaves in May, and wash with a Spunge with this Liquor Morning and Evening, and let it dry of itself.'
Charles Carter (cook to the Duke of Argyll), *The Compleat City and Country Cook*, 1732

John Parkinson also recommended 'garden spurge, broom, madder, rue, gention, scabious, betony, elecampane, the great hawkweed and lupin to cleanse the skinne from freckles, sunburn and wrinkles'. Spurge, however, is poisonous, nor would I recommend rue.

Bruises

These are very painful as well as disfiguring and the following remedies will help relieve the pain as well as lessen the discolouration.

Make a poultice of hyssop leaves. Allow to cool until tepid and apply to the bruise. Leave on for at least twenty minutes – longer if possible (for instructions on how to make a poultice, see p. 34).

Liquidize a tablespoon of parsley with a tablespoon of witch-hazel. Strain out the parsley residue through coffee filter paper and keep the mixture iced in the refrigerator. Pat it on to the bruise constantly throughout the day. If the bruise is also accompanied by swelling, soak a bandage in the mixture and wrap it round the bruise. Change the bandage and repeat the process once it has dried out. Keep this up until the swelling has subsided.

'The roote of Solomon's Seal – stamped while it is fresh and greene, and applied, taketh away in one night or two at the most, any bruse, blacke or blew spots gotten by fals or women's wilfulness, in stumbling upon their hasty husband's fists or such like.'

John Gerard, *The Herball and Generall Historie of Plants*, 1597

A unique way of acquiring a bruise, perhaps, but the pulverized root of Solomon's seal does work, though I found it took three days to clear the bruise.

Thread Veins

Thread veins are a complaint delicate English complexions seem particularly prone to. Not surprisingly, old English recipes seem to have discovered the best way of dealing with them. The first golden rule is to avoid making them worse by doing the sort of things that started them in the first place. The tiny network of broken veins just beneath the surface of the skin is caused by exposing unprotected skin to sudden harsh changes in temperature. This is particularly true during the winter when people rush from heated rooms into the cold outdoors, pushing the blood up to the surface of the skin with enormous force. So always protect your skin from the elements with a moisturizer, never use an astringent containing any alcohol, and wrap up warmly in the winter protecting as much of your face as you can with big woolly hats and scarves. Coffee, tea, alcohol, excessively smoky rooms and very spicy foods all help to dilate thread veins and make them worse. I am not suggesting you give up all these delights and live the life of a hermit, just that you partake of them in moderation. Drink very weak coffee, avoid spirits and stick to the odd glass of wine and drink herbal teas. Chamomile, yarrow and coltsfoot are particularly helpful taken internally. Never use a facial steam or subject your skin to alternate splashes of hot and cold water. Instead bathe the face twice daily in lukewarm infusions of coltsfoot tea. Tone the skin with chamomile tea or marigold milk.

Marigold Milk

Infuse 30 g (1 oz) of marigolds in half a litre (18 fl oz) of milk for twelve hours. Strain out the marigold. Keep the lotion cool but not refrigerated and be generous with it. Then apply lots and lots of the following moisturizer:

Marigold Moisturizer

45 g (1½ oz) anhydrous lanolin

120 ml (4 fl oz) wheatgerm oil

30 ml (1 fl oz) of an infusion made from 20 g (⅔ oz) of marigolds and 20 g (⅔ oz) of coltsfoot infused in 4 cups of water (save any spare infusion for use as a compress with which to dab the thread veins)

3 drops essential oil of marigold

Follow the Basic Cream Directions (p. 57). 120 ml of wheatgerm oil may seem excessive but wheatgerm is particularly soothing and healing for this condition.

Centuries ago, when smallpox was prevalent and the scars were a problem, people used to apply poultices of marigold petals twice daily to heal and gradually remove the scars over a period of time. This cream, if used continually for three to six months, will gradually help to fade and may even finally obliterate scars.

Sunburn

If I tell you exactly what happens to your skin when you tan it may put you off for ever or, failing that, at least I hope it will remind you to approach the sun with caution.

Tanning is caused by the ultra-violet rays of the sun in the burning range. To combat these your skin churns out melanin. This darkens the skin, at the same time causing it to thicken, and it is this last effect which is the skin's major protection against burning.

Now let me toll the knell of doom. Exposure to the sun causes permanent irreversible damage to the skin. Apart from ageing it, drying it up and encouraging thread veins it heightens one's susceptibility to skin cancer. A sample of skin taken from the bottom of an eighty-year-old man compared favourably to skin samples taken from a baby, whereas skin taken from any other part of his body looked like what it was – eighty-year-old skin. The moral of that tale being that the elderly gent's bottom was one part of his anatomy which hardly ever saw the sun and so remained baby-smooth. So sunbathe with caution. Sunbathing in the nude is not a good idea as parts which are generally not exposed to the sun burn very quickly. Step up your intake of vitamin B complex and vitamin C, which the sun depletes while you are tanning. If you simply must acquire a sun-tan here are some recipes which will help you look after your skin while you do so.

Sesame and Wheatgerm Tanning Oil

Sesame oil absorbs the ultra-violet rays of the sun more fully than any other natural oil. However, it is very greasy and water-resistant, so mix it up half-and-half with coconut oil or almond oil and use a teaspoon of wheatgerm oil and a few drops of iodine. This is particularly good for skin that takes a tan well. If you decide to use coconut oil remember to melt it down first. Once amalgamated it may thicken the whole mixture, but it should not turn it solid. If it does, simply leave the bottle on a warm beach or in the airing cupboard overnight before applying.

Marshmallow Cream (for more sensitive skins)

15 g (½ oz) anhydrous lanolin

15 g (½ oz) cocoa butter

70 ml (2⅓ fl oz) sesame oil

20 ml (⅔ fl oz or 4 tsp) wheatgerm oil

30 ml (1 fl oz) decoction of marshmallow root

30 ml (1 fl oz) infusion of violet flowers

6 drops iodine

3 drops essential oil of bergamot or lavender

Follow the Basic Lotion Directions (p. 58). The essential oils will help discourage midges, and bergamot oil, used in moderation, helps accelerate the tanning process. More than the specified amounts may lead to burning and a blotchy tan, so don't overdo it.

Apply tan creams and oils liberally, not forgetting to spread them on your ears, under your eyes, on your neck, and on the soles of your feet. Wear a good pair of sun glasses to protect your eyes from high intensities of ultra-violet light, which tires them and hurts them.

If after all my warnings you have made yourself look like the Sunday joint do two things: drink lots of cold water and apply one of the following remedies liberally to the sore bits.

Remedies to Take the Sting and the Pain out of Sunburn

Slices of cucumber rubbed on to the skin or cucumber juice

patted on the skin. To extract the juice from a cucumber chop it up into cubes. Do not remove the skin. Put it into a liquidizer with a few tablespoons of water. Liquidize. Strain through coffee filter paper.

Strong cold tea.

Live plain yoghurt. Messy, smelly but effective, as I discovered, guided by the advice of an old Greek lady.

Neat cider vinegar. It stings but very quickly takes away the pain.

The juice of houseleek rubbed on to the skin. This is especially helpful if you only have a small burnt place, such as your nose.

Make a decoction of quince seeds by boiling 15 g (½ oz) in a litre (1¾ pints) of water, for fifteen minutes. Strain. Soak pieces of surgical gauze in the decoction and spread these over the burnt areas. As soon as they begin to dry remove them, resoak, re-apply. Keep up this routine until the pain from the sunburn has lessened considerably.

Double-strength decoctions of any of the following herbs:

chamomile
comfrey leaves
marshmallow root
sage
St John's wort

Witchhazel, diluted with water 1:2, and combined with a teaspoon of cider vinegar. Use this last remedy only on naturally darker skins.

Exfoliation using cereal scrubs helps to remove the last of a fading jaundiced tan, as do all the remedies for freckles, while cowslip petals mashed into yoghurt and used as a face pack whiten the skin. Some old fashioned remedies for sunburn worked, others didn't.

A remedy y^t ye Sunne shall not hurt you shining on your head
'If you put a little branch of penny Royall in each eare ye sun will never make your head ache with shining on you.'

Sloane MS. 2552

Rampant superstition, I am afraid. You would be better off with a hat. But the following old recipe does work:

'That all the body maybe of a clear and glad and bright hue, take oil and dregs of old wine equally much, put them in a mortar,

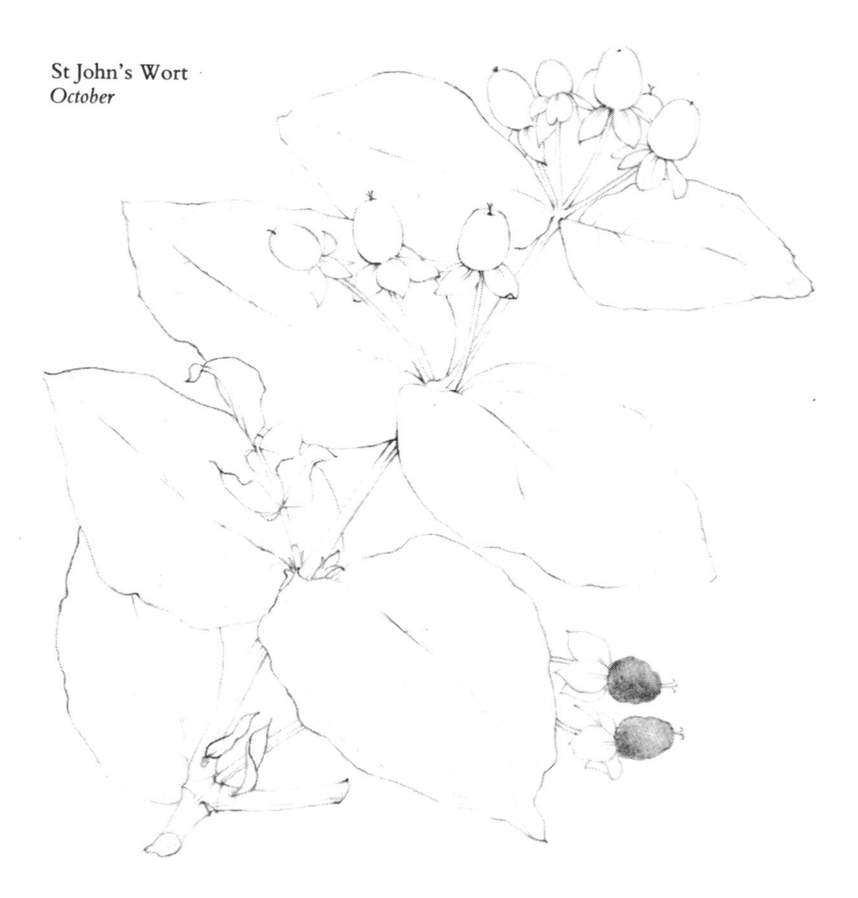

St John's Wort
October

mingle well together, and smear the body with this in the sun.'

The Anglo-Saxon *Leech Book of Bald*, A.D. 900–950

The *Leech Book of Bald* is the oldest existing herbal in England – any earlier herbals were probably destroyed in the course of the Viking invasion, when so many valuable monastic libraries were razed to the ground. It is particularly interesting because of the remarkably wide knowledge of herbs it exhibited which outstripped even the expertise of the doctors of Salerno, the oldest medical school in Europe. Unlike all the other scientific theses written at the time almost all of it is written in the vernacular, Anglo-Saxon. Latin only crops up in the text rarely. The 109 vellum leaves were written by a scribe (Cild) for Bald, a leech or herbalist, although two other leeches (Dun and Oxa), are mentioned as contributing prescriptions.

Herpes

These weeping cold sores or blisters which usually appear round the mouth can be helped with better nutrition, less stress and protection of the mouth from the sun with a zinc-oxide cream or a sun barrier lipsil. Some people find dabbing on a tincture of camphor at the first sign of a swelling helpful. Personally I find this too strong and prefer dabbing the incipient sore with horseradish milk, (see section on eczema, p. 170). Other helpful dabs include finely grated raw apple, fresh lemon juice, birch milk, a double-strength infusion of sage and live plain yoghurt, which is especially good for soothing dry, cracked cold sores.

Herbal Cold Sore Lotion

30 g (1 oz) elecampane root

30 g (1 oz) marshmallow root

30 g (1 oz) comfrey root

6 drops tincture of myrrh

Barely cover the roots with water and boil in a partly covered enamel saucepan for twenty minutes or until the liquid is reduced by half. Strain out the herbs and add the tincture of myrrh. Use the residue of herbs as a poultice for the sore. As often as you can during the day dab the liquid on the cold sore. As long as the cold sore lasts, treat it internally by eating five sorrel leaves chopped into a salad daily.

Chapped and Peeling Lips

The indelible dyes contained in some lipsticks may be making the problem worse because such dyes are photosensitive and cause cracking, drying and peeling. So try and find out exactly what is in your lipstick, and, if in doubt, throw it out. Chapped lips can be helped by mixing two drops of essential oil of sage with half a teaspoon of clear honey and spreading it on to the lips before you go to bed.

Lip Salve

30 g (1 oz) beeswax

30 ml (1 fl oz) apricot oil

30 ml (1 fl oz) wheatgerm oil

3 drops lavender oil

Melt the apricot and wheatgerm oils and the wax together and continue stirring while the mixture cools. Add the lavender oil when it is lukewarm and stir it in thoroughly. If you do not like the taste of lavender oil try the following recipe which is very pleasant tasting:

To Make Lipp Salve
'Take 6 spoonfuls of Sallet Oyle, put into it as much beeswax as ye quantity of 2 great nutmegs, 3 raisins of ye Sun Stoned and Slit, melt all them together on ye fire stirring it with a Sprigg of Rosemary and put in as much fine Sugar as will lie upon 3 pence, when it is all melted together put it into a gally pot. You may if you

please put in a spoonful of Rosewater in ye bottom of a Porringer, when you goe to melt it for your use.'

Mary Doggett, *Book of Receipts*, 1682

I took '3 pence' to mean something approximately the size of one of our old English sixpences which are still in circulation and now worth 2½p. When I make up this recipe I use teaspoonfuls as 'spoonfuls' and select chunks of beeswax as near as possible to the size of two large nutmegs. I use muscatel raisins and fine brown sugar and add the rose water to the mixture last, rather than before its use. This softens the salve which can then easily be applied with a fingertip. I store it in a large wide-necked jar and the result is definitely worth the effort. Not only is it effective but it tastes delicious. The Jacobeans would have stored this mixture in a small earthenware glazed pot, usually used by an apothecary.

Chapter 8
Tranquillity without Tranquillizers

Stress comes from a number of sources but there is no doubt that modern society, with its accent on pace, achievement and aggression, bombards the mind and body with stimuli which induce nervous tension, irritability, muscular aches, stomach disorders, acute depression and phobias. Stress can also wreak havoc on the body externally, producing skin eruptions, lesions, rashes and specific skin diseases such as furnunculosis, psoriasis, acne, eczema and herpes. Nothing is more ageing than constant worry. The antithesis – a relaxed emotional and mental attitude – works wonders for the exterior.

Facts About Stress

Modern society certainly does not have a monopoly of stress. Old herbals bulge with prescriptions intended to combat 'spleene, melancholic, frantiquenes, trubellsum sleep, the mare and the hag'. But the facts about just how acute and widespread stress is today are enough to provoke anxiety all by themselves. In the United States of America 5,000 million pills a year are swallowed to soothe anxieties, counteract depression and induce sleep or wakefulness. In 1977 it was estimated that just over 60 per cent of the British population (children included) had at some time used psychotropic drugs – those drugs that alter mood, consciousness or behaviour. Even this frightening statistic fails to take into account the hundreds of millions of aspirins which are swallowed in an attempt to relieve stress-induced headaches and stomach upsets. In Britain this has reached the astronomical proportions of three tons daily. The abuse of aspirin and patent medicines containing aspirin causes more deaths yearly in Britain than heroin. Approximately 7,000 people a year in Britain are admitted to hospital suffering from internal bleeding through taking aspirins, and of these unfortunates nearly 250 die.

Yet simple things like headaches can be treated quite effectively by herbs. Our Victorian grandmothers used to relieve their nervous headaches by pinning a sprig of lavender under the brim of their hats or drinking teas made of lavender or violet leaves. I am not suggesting that aspirin does not have a valuable place in medical treatment, and synthetic aspirin is certainly more effective than its forerunner the salicylic acid, derived directly from the willow, which tastes unpleasantly bitter and tends to irritate the stomach. But in many instances herbal methods of treatment are just as effective as their more stringent synthetic counterparts and have the added advantage of having no side-effects. They are also freely available and inexpensive.

It is not tobacco, coffee, tea, soft water or cholesterol but anxiety that is the biggest killer in the western world. One of the contributing factors to this problem is the philosophy behind modern medicine which divides symptoms, anatomy and personality (if it takes the latter into account at all) into tight, separate, airless compartments. Two thousand years ago Plato suggested a much more sympathetic, well-rounded approach to medicine when he wrote:

The cure of the part should not be attempted without treatment of the whole, and also no attempt should be made to cure the body without the soul, and therefore if the head and body are to be well you must begin by curing the mind: that is the first thing . . . For this is the great error of our day in the treatment of the human body, that physicians separate the soul from the body.

Plato, *Chronicles 156 e*

The beauty of herbal treatments is that they can be used to treat the whole body, internally and externally, and many herbs are definitely useful for nervous and psychological ailments. Every herb contains certain constituents which are peculiar to itself or its plant type, as well as common to many herbs. They contain vitamins, minerals, salts, acids, glycosides, tannins, mucilage, alkaloids and saponins. The minerals, acids and salts in herbs help the body resist disease, strengthen tissues and help to regulate the nervous system. The glycosides in herbs are broken down by fermentation and produce sugar and various compounds which contribute to the healthy functioning of the heart. Tannins help the body to recover from infection by blocking the passage of harmful bacteria. Mucilage is the slimier part of the fleshier herbs which covers the mucous membranes, protecting them and allowing them to heal. It also acts as a gentle laxative. It is not surprising, therefore, that many herbs, if included in your daily diet, will act as a tonic for your system, improving your general condition.

I am certainly not belittling the benefits of modern medicine (for our ancestors had little else to grasp at but herbal medicines and died like flies from infection and disease), but do try the walking-stick of herbal medicine before resorting to the wheelchair of modern allopathic medicine. You may well find the stick's modicum of gentle support is all you need to help you sleep soundly, to relieve the aches brought on by tension; to calm you or revive your flagging spirits.

Diet as a Way to Alleviate Stress

Eating wholefood, that is natural, unprocessed fresh foods, will ensure the supply of nutrients your system needs and lessen the risk of hypoglycaemia, the low blood glucose/sugar level which can result from a junk food diet relying heavily on white sugar. Many people will already be familiar with its symptoms – fatigue, depression and irritability – without knowing the specific cause of them. Of course, all our cells need some glucose sugar in order to function properly but, ironically, because of our present vastly increased consumption of sugar, refined carbohydrate and starchy food, hypoglycaemia has in fact become more common.

Thc rcason is simple. Refined white sugar is present in nearly every convenience food we eat. Even items you would not suspect, like frozen and tinned vegetables, contain sugar. White sugar penetrates through the walls of the stomach without first being digested and can create a state of imbalance in the calcium–phosphorus ratio in the body. It actually damages the natural blood sugar of the body and can facilitate the development of disorders of the pancreas and the nervous system.

So in the middle of the afternoon when you seize a great sticky bun and wash it down with a heavily sugared cup of tea in order to perk you up and give you the energy to get going again, you may well feel full of life, but the effect is fleeting and you will quickly succumb to tiredness and irritability again. Keep this unwise eating up and your nervous system will soon be crying out for something to calm it down.

Better energy producers can be found in the natural sugar contained in dried fruits and, of course, in honey. In addition to being a powerful antiseptic honey also contains mineral salts and vitamins C, E and A. What better way to take it, if you do not want to eat it straight off the spoon, than in milk and herbal teas? The warm mug of milk you may have been offered as a child really does help you sleep. Adelle Davis describes calcium as being as soothing as a mother, as relaxing as a sedative and as life-saving as an oxygen tent. Milk is an excellent source of mineral calcium which soothes the nerves and helps the relaxation because it helps the transportation of nerve impulses. If you lack calcium you cannot absorb enough vitamin C, and calcium deficiency results in tension, irritability, insomnia and indigestion. People who suffer from a build-up of nervousness and tension before performing in public or taking part in some competitive sport are well-advised to increase the calcium in their diet. I have to give many lectures, interviews and make numerous public appearances in the course of my work and somehow I have never managed to relax sufficiently to classify myself as an old hand at the business. So on any day when I know I have to make a public appearance (and television scares me particularly) I make sure I deliberately step up my calcium content with a dandelion salad or chamomile or nettle tea. There are many other excellent herbal sources of calcium (see p. 43).

Everything that applies to calcium applies to magnesium as well. Magnesium has been described as nature's own tranquillizer and in general you need only half as much magnesium as calcium to ensure the balance that will protect your nervous system – 400 mg of magnesium and 1 g of calcium. This is important because although it would be difficult for you to have too much magnesium if you decided to be a fanatic about it excessive quantities will act as a depressant. Herbs rich in magnesium are bladderwrack, devil's bit, dandelion leaves, kale, kelp, meadowsweet, mistletoe, great mullein leaves, parsley, peppermint, primrose, silverweed, walnut leaves and wintergreen.

Vitamin B complex is particularly important for energy and strong nervous reflexes. Vitamin B_6, or pyridoxine, is essential if the brain is to function correctly. Recent studies have shown that many women suffering from severe depression while on the pill (I cannot say 'because of the pill' as this has not been conclusively proved) have improved enormously after taking controlled doses of vitamin B_6. But this vitamin cannot be properly absorbed unless magnesium is present. Vitamin B_6 is present in yeast, black strap molasses, wheatbran, wheatgerm and kidneys and liver. Unhappily, alcohol is lethal to vitamin B: put all these good sources of vitamin B in your body and follow them with a heavy drinking session and you will emerge not just with a furry tongue and a hangover, but totally robbed of all the energy vitamin B gives you.

The way in which you eat your food is just as important as what you eat. Eating meals on the run, standing up, crouched over your office desk or, worse still, missing them out altogether will almost certainly, if you keep it up, result in indigestion at best or at worst in severe stomach disorders and the inability of the digestive tract to absorb and use whatever nourishment you might be pushing its way. Tension slows down digestion and inhibits the manufacture of hydrochloric acid and other digestive fluids so food cannot be assimilated. So try, if you can, to eat your food in congenial surroundings which make you feel relaxed, comfortable and happy and, above all, which please *you* – that's the important thing. A restaurant with pink tablecloths, soft candlelight and deferential waiters might be just the thing to relax some people and make others feel so uneasy that they finish with acute indigestion. Try to eat slowly. This will bring the added pleasure of actually being able to taste your food and allow for the more mundane necessity of chewing it thoroughly and so will help the first step to its digestion.

When Hippocrates said 'let food be your medicine and medicine your food', he was advising his fellow Greeks about the use of herbs. Certain herbs included in your diet in the form of teas, green milks, wines, liqueurs or added to bread, scones, desserts, sauces, salads and cooked dishes, can all help to alleviate stress which may appear as anxiety, tension, insomnia, hysteria, depression, high blood pressure, migraine, headaches and skin disturbances. The following list of herbs does not claim to be comprehensive. Firstly, I do not want to overwhelm you with choice (which could lead to all sorts of anxieties about the choosing) and secondly, I prefer to recommend only herbs I have had some dealings with. Where it is particularly important to measure out the herb carefully or to use only a certain part of the herb I have stated this, as some herbs like mistletoe and valerian are particularly strong. Do not get carried away with the idea that all herbs are gentle in their effect. It is true that most herbal treatments will not produce immediate and spectacular cures; their effect is gentle and cumulative. But some herbs can, if taken unwisely in dosages which are too strong, produce vomiting, diarrhoea, headaches, dizziness or stomach pains which, though not fatal, can be unpleasant, painful and which anyway are entirely unnecessary if you follow my instructions to the letter wherever I have given specific doses.

Rather than listing herbs alphabetically it is more useful to group them together under the name of the condition they alleviate. But it must be understood that because every herb contains so many different properties, a single herb may help with many conditions, both internal and external. Some herbs help several complaints and herbs such as nettles, sage and vervain are 'cure alls', that is, their effect on the whole body and the mind is so widespread that they act as a general tonic.

Herbs Which Are Believed to be Cheering and Which Are General Tonics

Borage contains potassium, calcium and various acids, and it is these constituents, which may be extracted from its fresh juice, that provide its invigorating properties. I have given a few excellent summer parties with the help of the following cider cup containing borage, and have seen my guests leaving decidedly exhilarated.

Cider Cup

2 litres (4 pints) dry cider
½ litre (1 pint) pineapple juice
½ litre (1 pint) orange juice
1 glass sherry
dash of Angostura bitters
ice
3 sprigs lemon balm
6 young borage leaves

Place all the ingredients, except the ice, balm and borage, in a large bowl and mix thoroughly. Liquidize the borage with the ice and add this mixture to the cider cup. Allow to stand for an hour before serving. Float the sprigs of balm on the top and once the cup is poured add a single borage flower stripped of its calyx floating face up to each glass. If you are feeling adventurous, the flowers can be eaten.

The borage leaves can also be used as part of a salad. Pick the tenderest young leaves at the top of the plant and while washing them in running water rub them gently to remove the white hairs which will only feel unpleasantly prickly if chewed. The flowers added to salads look beautiful but do remember to remove their hairy calyces first and scatter them over the top of the salad *after* you have dressed it with vinaigrette, otherwise they will emerge looking sad and battered by the dressing and the tossing. Flowers in salads may sound unorthodox but centuries ago salads were most elaborate affairs, sometimes containing as many as thirty ingredients, including many herbs we would never even consider using nowadays.

Nettles contain more iron than spinach does, together with valuable mineral salts and vitamin C, and they make an excellent general tonic. They are tastiest when gathered at their tenderest in the spring. Always wear gardening gloves, trousers and long sleeves when harvesting them. Wash them, shake off any excess water, strip the leaves off the stalk (still wearing protective gloves) and put in an enamel saucepan with a knob of butter. Cover the saucepan closely and sweat the nettles very gently over a low heat, shaking the pan occasionally so that they become evenly buttered. Add a sprinkling of sea salt, a touch of freshly ground black pepper and drain well in a fine-meshed nylon sieve (a metal sieve or colander will contaminate the delicate flavour of the nettles making them taste 'irony' and bitter). Add a squeeze of lemon juice, some freshly chopped chives, another knob of butter and serve. Save the strained-off juices as stock for vegetable soup. Never pick nettles which have gone to seed. They taste very bitter and unpleasant.

Nettle tea can be made successfully with fresh or dried leaves. Use four fresh nettle tops about 10 cm (4 in.) long added to a litre (1 ¾ pints) of boiling water, or take 20 g (⅔ oz) of the dried leaves for the same quantity of water. If you make the tea any stronger than this, you will get an uncomfortable burning sensation in your mouth which may spread to the rest of your body. It is a decidedly unpleasant feeling, so follow the quantities given carefully. Drink the tea with a slice of lemon and some honey.

Sage. The Chinese have always been amazed that we should be foolish enough to import tea from them when we have sage here. The Dutch, being wise traders and good businessmen, used to export 1 lb of dried sage to China in return for every 4 lb of China tea. Sage has long had a reputation for restoring and maintaining health. It is another 'cure all'.

I often make sage bread for lunch and serve it hot out of the oven with robust English cheeses such as Cheddar and Double Gloucester.

Sage Bread

15 g (½ oz) fresh yeast or 2 level tsp dried yeast

3 tbsp warm water

1 dessertspoon brown muscovado sugar

¼ kilo (½ lb) wholemeal flour

¼ kilo (½ lb) strong white flour

2 dessertspoons dried sage

1 tsp allspice, crushed

1 tsp celery seed

30 g (1 oz) melted butter

300 ml (10 fl oz) warm milk

1 beaten egg

sesame seeds

Dissolve the yeast in the warm water with the sugar and leave in a warm place for ten minutes, until it foams. Meanwhile, put the two flours, sage, salt, celery seed and spice into a large bowl. Pour in the warm milk, melted butter, beaten egg and the yeast. Mix with a wooden spoon (as the mixture is stiff and difficult to handle, I find a spoon with a long handle helps here). Knead on a floured board until the dough feels elastic and stops sticking to the board. Put back into the bowl and cover with a damp cloth. Leave to rise in a warm place for half an hour. Turn out and knead again until the dough stops sticking to the board and feels light and malleable. Shape into a plaited loaf and leave to rise again. To make a plaited loaf cut the dough into three equal-sized pieces. Shape each piece into a long thin roll and plait together. Fold under the ends. Splash the top of loaf with a little milk and sprinkle liberally with sesame seeds. Bake for half an hour at gas mark 7 or 220°C (425°F).

Herbal Tranquillizers

Vervain is believed to be especially good for relieving the sort of prolonged mental stress which may show itself as constant severe headaches as well as tension in the neck and shoulders.

Vervain Bath

Add 200 g (7 oz) of dried vervain leaves to 2 litres (3½ pints) of cold water. Bring to the boil then immediately remove from the stove. Leave to brew for fifteen minutes. Strain through a nylon sieve into your warm bath water. This makes a most refreshing bath, soothing away tension, especially round the neck and shoulders, so be sure to immerse yourself thoroughly in the water putting a folded towel draped over the edge of the bath on which to rest your head. The towel will provide the extra grip you need to prevent yourself from slipping under the water altogether! Vervain can also be drunk as a tea. Make a decoction using 50 g (1¾ oz) to a litre (1¾ pints) of water. This can be drunk last thing at night to encourage sound sleep.

Alternatively, soak a flannel in the tea and apply it to the forehead and temples to soothe away headaches. A flannel and small towel immersed in the same tea, slightly wrung out and draped round the neck and shoulders will also soothe away tension in this area, but do keep both yourself and the tea warm while you carry out this treatment, otherwise you will finish up with magnificently tension-free shoulders and severe rheumatism.

Woodruff is a natural tranquillizer which soothes, calms, relaxes and is especially good for people suffering from extreme nervous tension which prevents them sleeping. The leaves only exude their inimitable odour redolent of new-mown hay and honey with a hint of vanilla once they are dry, so this fragrant herb can be used to stuff pillows. Alternatively, keep muslin sachets of woodruff permanently in your linen cupboard to scent all your sheets. The fragrance will last even once the sheets have been on the bed for two or three days. I have always found woodruff a much more satisfactory sleep-inducing herb than hops.

The dried leaves impart a lovely subtle flavour to the following German wine cup:

Maibowle

2 bottles medium dry white wine

thinly peeled shreds of lemon rind

¼ kilo (½ lb) hulled strawberries, sliced in half

5 sprigs dried woodruff

juice of 1 lemon

clear honey to taste

2 bottles tonic water

spearmint

borage flowers

First put as many glasses as you will need in the coldest part of the fridge to chill. Lightly crush the dried woodruff and put into a very large jug or bowl with half a bottle of wine. Steep for an hour. Remove the sprigs of woodruff and add all the remaining ingredients except the mint and borage flowers. Take the iced glasses out of the fridge, add a mint sprig to each, pour in the wine cup and float a borage flower face up in each glass.

Herbs Which Help Relieve Extreme Fatigue and Insomnia

Lemon Balm was recommended by Coghan as:

'An herbe greatly to be esteemed of Studentes. For that by a special propertie, it driveth away heavinesse of minde, sharpneth the understanding and the wit, and encreaseth memorie.'

Thomas Coghan, *The Haven of Health; chiefly gathered for the comfort of Students, and consequently of all those that have a care of their health*, 1584

Lemon balm is less exhilarating than borage but I find it extremely good for insomnia and nervous headaches.

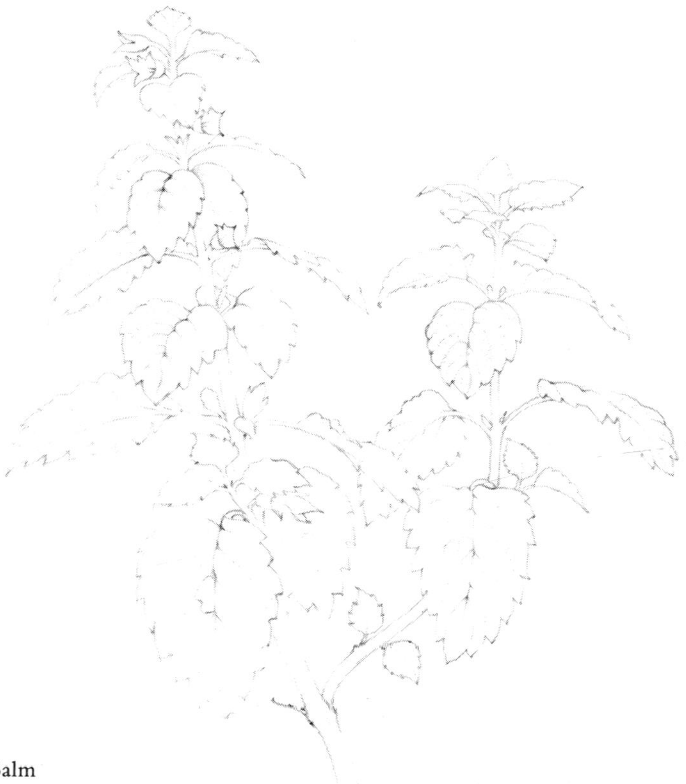

Lemon Balm
September

Carmelite water was originally distilled by monks and nuns and was dabbed on the forehead to relieve nervous headaches. *The London Dispensatory* of 1696 suggested the water would 'cure baldness and renew youth' though whether the youth would be part of the psychological bonus of renewed hair growth is a moot point.

Carmelite Water

240 g (8 oz) balm leaves

30 g (1 oz) lemon peel, coarsely grated

½ litre (1 pint) orange flower water

2 tbsp nutmeg, grated

2 tbsp coriander seeds

2 tbsp cloves

1 tsp cinnamon sticks

1 tsp dried angelica root

1 litre (1¾ pints) vodka

Lightly crush the first seven ingredients in a mortar. Put these together with the orange flower water and vodka in a teapot still. Distil slowly, strain off, bottle and stopper or cap the bottles tightly. The fragrance tends to get more subtle and mellower the longer the water is left to stand.

Balm tea is very simply made. Use 30 g (1 oz) of the fresh leaves to a litre (1¾ pints) of boiling water. Add a squeeze of lemon juice and a curl of lemon peel if you want to heighten the delicate lemony flavour and sweeten with a touch of honey. I drink this copiously in the summer but the dried leaves do not make a satisfactory winter tea. The finely shredded young leaves of balm are very palatable if strewed sparingly on green salads or salads of oranges and green olives and they can be mixed with cream cheese and a trace of garlic as a filling for wholemeal sandwiches. I also mix a little of the fragrant oil obtained from balm leaves with my furniture polish (it is the cream not the wax type). This gives anything you polish with it a lovely delicate lemony smell and I find the subtle pervasion of the fragrance throughout my house very cheering.

Chamomile. Common chamomile smells of apples and, in the Middle Ages, was used as one of the aromatic strewing herbs as well as for lawns. It seems to thrive on being trodden on, a fact that must have been well known in Shakespeare's time, for he has Falstaff say to Henry, Prince of Wales:

'Harry, I do not only marvel where thou spendest thy time, but

also how thou art accompanied. For though the camomile, the more it is trodden on, the faster it grows, yet youth, the more it is wasted the sooner it wears.'

Henry IV, Part I, Act II, Scene 4

The Elizabethans also used the dried leaves for smoking before the introduction of tobacco, believing the fragrance from the smoke helped sleeplessness.

A tea is less noxious and easier to make. Simply add 20 g (⅔ oz) of the flowers of common chamomile to a litre (1¾ pints) of freshly boiled water. Then cover tightly the vessel in which you are brewing the tea to stop the steam escaping – the medicinal value of the flowers is greatly impaired by any evaporation. Infuse for ten minutes, strain through a nylon sieve, sweeten with honey and stir with a long cinnamon stick which adds a subtle spicy flavour to the tea.

Parkinson recommended bathing in chamomile 'to strengthen the sound and to ease pains in the diseased'. You will need a lot of patience and some big saucepans for the following chamomile bath but, equipped with these two prerequisites, the results are well worth the effort.

Chamomile Bath

'To make a bath for Melancholy. Take Mallowes, pellitory of the wall, of each three handfuls, Camomell flowers, Mellilot flowers, of each one handfull, hollyhocks, two handfuls, Isop one greate handfull, senerick seed one ounce, and boil them in nine gallons of water until they come to three, then put in a quart of new milke and go into it bloude warme or something warmer.'

Mary Fairfax, *Still-Room Book*, 1630

I must admit I cheat a little. I do not have enough room on my stove to heat 9 gallons of water so I cut the original recipe by two-thirds. (This also means I have less of the resulting brew to carry upstairs!) I miss out the senerick seed as I have never been able to discover what it is but I do use all the other ingredients. 'Isop' is hyssop and pellitory of the wall is sometimes known as lichwort. The 'mellilot' is *Melilotus officinalis*, or sweet clover, which was much more common in the sixteenth century than it is now. As I have difficulty finding this herb I substitute red clover instead. It is perfectly alright to use the dried equivalent of the fresh herbs. If you are cutting the recipe by two-thirds, as I do, put 30 g (1 oz) of each herb into 16 litres (3 gallons) of water and add half a litre (1 pint) of milk.

Valerian root smells obnoxiously of stale perspiration, which is formed by oxidation of the essential oil which, once the root is exposed, turns into valerianic acid. Rats and cats love the

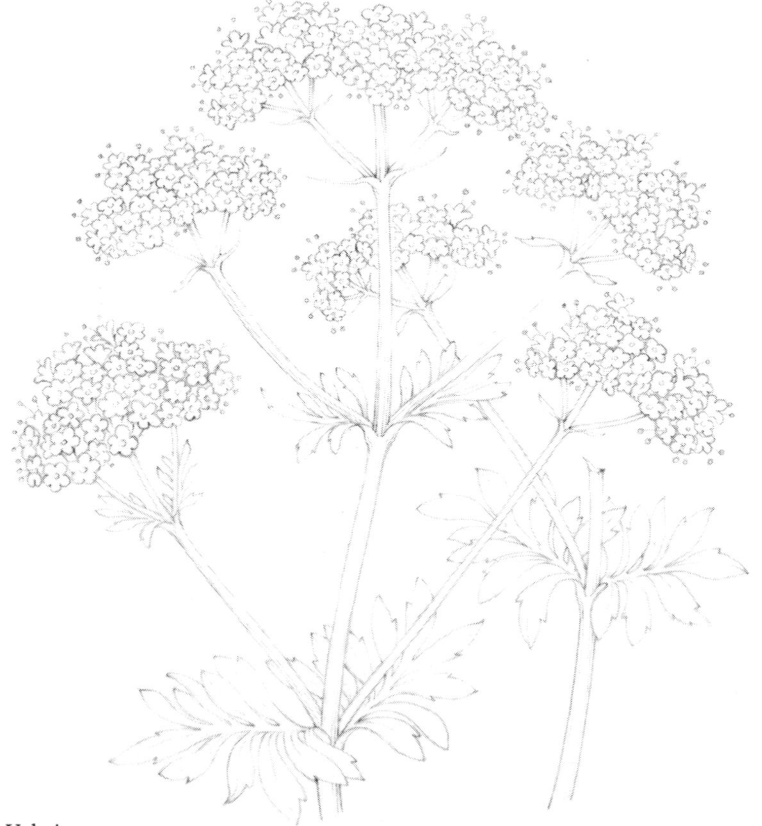

Valerian
August

smell. My own cat spends hours with her head down sniffing at the roots and trembling with delight. It has been suggested that the rat-attracting powers of the Pied Piper of Hamelin was the result of the bits of valerian root he secreted on his person.

It is the root that is mainly used to help relieve the sort of nervous exhaustion brought on by too much excitement which may result in palpitations, breathlessness, nervous contractions of the stomach or migraines. During the Second World War, valerian was given to people whose nerves had been stretched to breaking point by repeated air raids. It has none of the harmful after-effects produced by narcotics, but be warned: in over-large doses or doses which are repeated too often, it can cause severe headaches; mental agitation, delusions, heaviness, stupor; or, at the other extreme, restlessness. Properly used, valerian is certainly the supreme cure for all types of nervous complaints. Try to use the fresh root, which is of greater medicinal value than the dried and, as the roots are perennial, they should be allowed to be at least two years old before being dug up. Having removed all the earth from the root by washing it thoroughly, slice up a level tablespoon as finely as you can and pour over half a litre (1 pint) of water which has been brought to boiling point but not actually allowed to boil. This subtle differentiation is very important, for only slow, gentle heating should be used for the valerian root. Allow the tea to steep overnight. Strain and take two tablespoons a quarter of an hour before your three main daily meals. If insomnia is your problem take two tablespoons an hour or so before going to bed. As valerian tastes rather unpleasant, I usually have a teaspoon of raw honey standing by to mask it. Some people add a drop of peppermint or clove oil to the dose; I find this unpleasantly strong, though you may like to try it and see.

If you feel at all anxious about not getting the dosage of valerian correct it is possible to buy liquid extract of valerian from some of the more old-fashioned chemists. The dosage should be measured out with an eyedropper and is ten to fifteen drops in a glass of water nightly, although the chemist will write the dose that is correct for your needs on the label.

Red clover. It has long been noted that cattle seem particularly content when grazing in a clover field, hence the phrase 'living in clover'. I find clover tea, which is very pleasant to taste, excellent for stilling a carousel of anxious thoughts and so promoting sleep. Infuse 20 g (⅔ oz) of the fresh flowers in a litre (1¾ pints) of boiling water for ten minutes. Strain and sweeten, if possible with aromatic clover honey, which complements the delicate taste of the clover. Alternatively, a small number of flowers can be shredded in a salad and the salad can be dressed with a vinaigrette sweetened with clover honey.

Cowslip flowers contain narcotic juices and were believed to be particularly good for inducing sleep.

A Comfortable Cordial to Cause Sleep

'Take an ounce of Surrup of Cowslips and half an ounce of Gillyflowers, and a dram of Diascordium and a quarter of a pint of Cowslips water, and mix them altogether and so take a spoonful of it at a time.'

Egerton MS. 2415

Cowslip wine might prove more palatable. Be warned: if kept too long it can be highly intoxicating (here speaks the voice of experience).

Cowslip Wine

Collect a shoe-boxful of cowslip blossom, just the petals not the green calyx. Make sure they are all free of dirt and insects, washing if necessary under running water and shaking off any remaining droplets. Put the peel of two oranges and two lemons in a large saucepan and pour over 3 litres (5¼ pints) of boiling water in which 70 g (2⅓ oz) of honey has been dissolved. Cool then add the cowslip blossom. Cover and let stand for three days, stirring the mixture from time to time. Strain into fermentation jars and leave for two weeks until the fermentation has stopped. Close off tightly and leave undisturbed for four months. Syphon off, bottle and drink as quickly as you can after that.

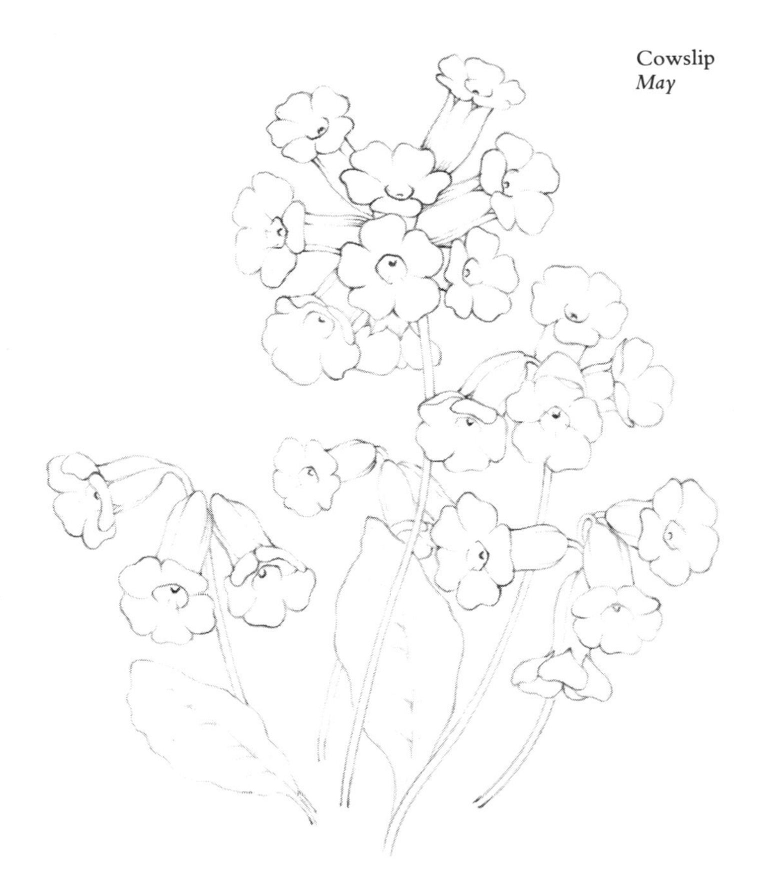

Cowslip
May

John Evelyn recommended the flowers pickled and added to salads, but I fear modern taste-buds would find the combination too sharp and vinegary. Try the young leaves roughly chopped as a milder, more acceptable substitute. They taste rather like watercress. By all means do not ignore the flowers. Scatter a few in a salad to add a splash of golden colour.

Hops, strangely enough, were first believed actually to encourage the onset of melancholy. John Evelyn did acknowledge that hops preserve beer but added 'they repay the pleasure in tormenting diseases and a shorter life'. But those of us who enjoy the odd pint of bitter need not be alarmed for it has since been discovered that the volatile oil in hops produces a soporific and sedative effect (as those of us who enjoy more than the odd few pints will already have discovered). An infusion of the hops' leaves and stalks in a litre (1¾ pints) of water will prove a soothing nightcap. I have found it less bitter and more palatable when mixed with equal parts of Earl Grey tea.

Hop pillows are said to induce sleep but they only seem to induce sneezes and running eyes with me. Consequently, my company does not sell hop pillows and, because of my preference, we use a traditional mixture of sleep herbs recommended by Mary Doggett in her receipt book of 1682 which includes lavender and rosemary. The mixture works for me and, judging by the number of letters I have had from customers and the fact that my staff have to leave the room every quarter of an hour when handling the mixture I gather it works for other people! A well-made herbal pillow should last for up to a year, after which time it can be refilled with a fresh mixture of herbs.

Herbs for Headaches

Lavender has been used for hundreds of years to alleviate headaches:

> 'Water of lavender hearbe and flowers chopped together and distilled in June is good against ye gyddynes of ye head.'
>
> Sloane MS. 10 Plut. IXXXIV.F.

I cannot recommend lavender too highly as a headache cure. A drop of lavender oil rubbed into each temple will work almost magically, but do be very sparing about the amount you use. Measure your lavender oil in drops: in large doses it is a narcotic poison. If that warning sounds like the knell of doom and has put you off using the oil, use lavender water instead. It can be splashed liberally on the forehead and temples and round the back of a tense aching neck. Culpeper was obviously aware of the dire effect the liberal use of lavender oil might have when he wrote 'the chymical oil drawn from Lavender usually called Oil of Spike, is of so fierce and piercing a quality that it is cautiously to be used, some few drops being sufficient to be given with other things, either for inward or outward griefs.' Lavender oil works wonders added to warm bath water if you are suffering from nervous exhaustion.

Lavender tea can also be used as a headache cure. Again, be careful about the quantities of lavender you add to the water to make the tea and never drink more than three cups a day. Add 10 g ($\frac{1}{3}$ oz) of the flowers to a litre ($1\frac{3}{4}$ pints) of boiling water, infuse for five minutes only, strain and drink. The taste takes a little getting used to.

Sweet violet. Sadly, violets are found increasingly rarely in woodlands and shady country lanes. Because of their increasing scarcity, you may need a description of the plant to identify it. Do not mistake it for the potted African variety which is altogether much larger and has very little fragrance. Wild violets have heart-shaped, velvety, dark green leaves and viola-shaped flowers, which range from white to deep purple. Considering the increasing scarcity of violets it would be as well to grow your own and not denude the countryside of those that are left. Many herb nurseries sell seedlings which will flourish in a damp sheltered corner of the garden.

Shakespeare in his inimitable observant way described the smell of violets as:

'Sweet, not lasting,
The perfume and suppliance of a minute, no more'

Hamlet, Act I, Scene 3

When I was a child I thought I could actually sniff the smell out of violets, for Shakespeare was absolutely right, after a few sniffs the smell apparently vanished so that, try as I might, I could not smell their fragrance any more. The explanation for this phenomenon is simple and sadly far less magical than my childhood conviction. Ionone is the dominant substance in the violet's fragrance and it has a soporific effect on our sense of smell, so that it is this that is actually exhausted, not the scent of the violets. The old herbalists may not have been conversant with this scientific explanation but they were certainly keenly aware of the soporific effects violets had on people.

A violet foot bath containing ten or twelve flowers encourages sleep. Leave the flowers floating in the water. Wrap up warmly, then wriggle your bare toes in the foot bath for at least fifteen minutes. This gentle exercise will relieve your aching feet as well as help to waft the fragrance of violets upwards to soothe you to sleep. I have also found slightly crushed violet leaves bound to forehead and temples by an old scarf an excellent remedy for headaches. I specify an old scarf because the juice from the violet leaves is very staining, but do not worry, it will not leave your forehead an indelible green. This treatment is best carried out in the privacy of your own home for obvious reasons.

Homer and Virgil recommended violets for moderating anger, allaying sleeplessness, and to comfort and strengthen the heart. An infusion of violet flowers is, in fact, very good for soothing restlessness and jagged nerves. Pour a litre ($1\frac{3}{4}$ pints) of boiling water over 80 g ($2\frac{2}{3}$ oz) of freshly picked violets. Infuse for twelve hours, strain out the leaves and drink a wine glassful cold every two hours. Make this infusion fresh every day, throwing out any left-overs from the previous day. This tea tastes very scented and rather pleasant but if you prefer a sweeter version try:

Syrup of Violets

Pick $\frac{1}{4}$ kilo ($\frac{1}{2}$ lb) of violet flowers. Make sure they are dirt- and insect-free, then pour a litre ($1\frac{3}{4}$ pints) of freshly boiled water over them. Cover tightly and infuse for twenty-four hours. Strain off the liquid through a double layer of muslin or, better still, coffee filter paper. Add double the liquid's weight of honey and simmer in a heavy bottomed saucepan over a low heat, skimming off any scum which rises to the surface with a silver or stainless steel spoon (a wooden one is clumsy and inefficient and an iron or aluminium one will contaminate the violets with its irony flavour). As soon as the mixture takes on the consistency of syrup, remove from the heat, pour into sterilized jars and cover with wax-paper and lids. Take two level teaspoons daily but, beware, this syrup is also mildly laxative, so do not make it a continual habit. This syrup, stored in the refrigerator, will last for several months.

Viper's bugloss may be used in much the same way as borage. Liquidize the young leaves with ice and add them to cool summer drinks or shred them into salads. A tea of the fresh leaves can be made by adding a heaped handful to a litre ($1\frac{3}{4}$ pints) of boiling water and is particularly good for helping to dispel nervous headaches.

Roses. Gerard recommended rose water as 'good for strengthening of the hart and refreshing of the spirits and likewise in all things that require a gentle cooling'. So, the next time you can feel your temperature rising dab some rose water on your forehead and treat yourself to a ten-minute rest in a darkened room. The combination of the rose water and the peace will help you emerge feeling fragrant, refreshed and soothed.

If you have a raging headache which is also making you feel slightly nauseous, try putting three drops of essential oil of roses on a lump of sugar and dissolving it slowly in your mouth. I find this quells the nausea as well as soothing the headache.

As you sip your cup of herbal tea or glass of milk at night build up a conscious picture of yourself, about how you want to look and feel: radiant, alive, enthusiastic, joyous. Nothing damages you so much physically and spiritually as stress. My ayah (African nanny) used to tuck me up at night and tell me that if I went to sleep with a smile on my face I would have sweet dreams. It worked. It may have worked simply because of suggestion but in this tranquillizer-ridden modern age sleep induced by harmless suggestion is surely preferable to the sort of sleep made possible by potentially dangerous synthetic products.

Chapter 9
Grow your own Herbs

I hope that by reading this book and by experimenting with the recipes in it you will acquire a healthier, more beautiful body and a more serene attitude to life. So much of my own inner quiet springs from the absorbing pleasure of cultivating a herb garden that I feel this enjoyment might be worth sharing with you.

Herbs are generally very tough and, once established, tend to romp away and look after themselves. They do have a few dislikes. The woody herbs can survive constant wind but most other herbs appreciate the protection of a wall, hedge or interwoven fence. A herb hedge such as rosemary, lavender or sage is ideal, though sage does tend to get woody and need replanting every three or four years. The Elizabethans were fond of box hedges but unfortunately these are ideal breeding places for slugs and snails. Tusser and other experienced Elizabethan gardeners used to combat them with toads, giving them their own sunshine shelters by tipping over flower pots, but this idea may not appeal to you. My own herb garden is sheltered by a wall. Those old-fashioned kitchen garden walls are ideal because they trap the heat inside the garden and discourage the intrusion of weeds from the outside.

Most herbs like plenty of sunshine, though a few such as parsley, chives, lovage, chervil, houseleek and all mints except pennyroyal enjoy moist, partly sheltered sites. Herbs dislike being planted near voracious tree roots which rob them of valuable nutrients and make them grow tall, thin and straggly. In my ignorance I twice tried to plant seedlings of lady's mantle about 3 feet away from an old pear tree and they perished miserably. The advisory horticulturist of the Herb

Society told me he had a pear tree from a neighbouring garden leaning into his herb garden and he made a special point of picking up the fallen leaves daily before they could do any harm. In his experience they deterred the growth of the plants nearby. This may have been the problem with my lady's mantle which has since reseeded itself some 10 yards away from the pear tree and seems to be flourishing.

Soil

Most herbs like light soil, and a cover of garden peat spread 2½ cm (1 in.) thick keeps the soil friable and actually saves you weeding by keeping the soil underneath dark. Better still, it is hardly ever necessary to water the herb garden once it has good peat cover. Peat prevents the soil from cracking up with a sudden temperature change or from becoming waterlogged. Crumbly dark soil also encourages root growth. It should be applied in spring just after a light shower. Dampen it a little before spreading. Do not overfeed the soil with those instant chemical liquid and dissolvable powder fertilizers. Few herbs need much feeding and any nutrient they do need should be organic. Remember that many of the aromatic herbs originated in sunny Mediterranean or eastern countries which have little rain and soil that is not particularly rich. Over-fertilizing produces lush growth which reduces the aroma and the nutritive quality of the herb, but the judicious use of natural fertilizers will not upset the delicate balance of the powerhouse of minerals and vitamins which are present in every herb. Some herbs thrive only in a particular type of soil. My viper's bugloss, for example, could not adapt to the soil in my garden which is mostly loam. It looked as if it was about to die until a friend brought a big bag of the chalky soil from the South Downs where she had been on holiday. We replanted it and it is now flourishing.

Natural Fertilizers and Natural Fungal and Insect Repellents

Make the exclusive use of organic fertilizers and natural insect repellents the first unbreakable rule of your herb garden. You may well be tempted by the enormous range of chemical herbicides and pesticides available on the market but remember you are not growing herbs, like leeks, for their size so you can win prizes. The herbs richest in essential oils, minerals and vitamins are often the smallest and most unprepossessing. Nor do I feel that the chemicals used in repellent fertilizers have been tested long enough for us to be able to assess the damage these preparations might do. Keep your herbs chemical-free: the fewer chemicals you eat and put on your skin the better.

You can make your own organic fertilizers quite easily (and not only save bombarding your body with chemicals but ease the strain on your purse). This way you won't even have to invest in peat because the regular dressing of organic compost lightly forked into the soil and a 2½ cm (1 in.) layer left on top duplicates the natural conditions under which herbs grow best. If you have an elderberry bush or a birch tree this is the ideal site for a compost heap as the excretions from their roots, together with their fallen leaves, speed up fermentation, producing a light compost which is especially effective for revitalizing the soil. An efficient heap should measure 180 cm (6 ft) by 120 cm (4 ft) and should be enclosed by a fence of planks or wire netting fastened to stakes in the ground which is then lined with straw and sheets of newspaper. These will rot into the heap themselves and so will need renewing occasionally. The idea is to prevent currents of air keeping the margins cool. The heap should have its bottom firmly planted on the bare earth in order to admit the necessary soil bacteria which decomposes the waste. One side of the heap should have movable supports so that you can get at your compost.

If you have a small garden you may find it far more economical in terms of space to buy one of those bins specially designed for rotting waste into compost. I find them rather efficient. Either way you can build up an amazing cocktail of waste, weeds, leaves, lawn mowings uncontaminated with chemical weed killers, twigs, newspaper, vacuum cleaner dust, feathers, bits of cat and dog fluff, hay, straw, raw or cooked left-over food as well as other kitchen waste such as egg shells, vegetable peelings and discarded parts of raw fish. Spread these items 10 cm (4 in.) to 15 cm (6 in.) thick, sandwich with thinner layers of soil garnished with sprigs of the odd aromatic herb. Add a little herbal activator like stinging nettles, which are particularly good for helping the nitrogen bacteria break up decaying vegetable matter and the carbons which are present in paper. You can also use one made from seaweed. Comfrey, with its high calcium and nitrogen content, is a good enricher and yarrow added in minute quantities helps to speed up the process of decomposition. Use only two leaves finely shredded and well mixed into the heap – larger quantities do not accelerate the process still further, so do not go overboard with enthusiasm. Chamomile stops excessive acidification and will keep your compost heap sweet. Valerian flowers will stimulate the phosphorus activity in the heap; tansy adds invaluable potassium and the despised dandelion is full of minerals. All these herbs can be added fresh or dried to your compost heap, but do not add the roots, as generally they prove very difficult to break down. When the heap is 120 cm (4 ft) high put a lid of soil on it. The results will soon look like dark crumbly, appetizing Christmas pudding and your herbs can enjoy this festive food all year round. It seems crazy that amateur gardeners should be willing to spend 14 million pounds a year on fertilizers in at attempt to improve the soil structure when each household discards on average 2½ kilos of food and 6 kilos of waste paper weekly. I am aware that there are many other effective ways of making compost, but I have described the method I have found best for myself.

However, if you have not got the time to enjoy all this garden cookery use organic fertilizer like Biohumus or a seaweed preparation. Horsetail spray is quick to make and protects against fungus attacks as well as proving an excellent fertilizer. Horsetail's persistence may be the bane of tidy gardeners but it is an invaluable garden nurse.

Horsetail Fertilizer and Fungal Repellent

Horsetail looks rather like tatty thin asparagus with no leaves but with scaly sheaths projecting from the joints. Most people consider it a nuisance and regard it as a weed. It is, in fact, a valuable herb and grows wild. In May it produces little shoots which look like prehistoric miniature pine trees and these are the parts that should be used fresh or dry as a fertilizer. Cover 45 g (1½ oz) of dried or a generous handful of fresh horsetail with 6 litres (10 pints) of cold water. Bring slowly to the boil and simmer for twenty minutes. Take off the heat, cover tightly and leave to cool. Strain out the bits and use to spray your herbs until the foliage drips. Water the roots with whatever is left over.

This is particularly good for preventing mint rust and mildew and for deterring black spot on roses. It also gives drooping newly planted seedlings some backbone as it has abundant quantities of cobalt, calcium and silicon. I have found it especially useful for aromatic herbs newly planted in a rockery; they need a great deal of liquid attention for the first few weeks to minimize the baking effect of the sun on the rocks. It is also an excellent remedy for a herb suspected of having a root disease.

Nettles abound in nitrogen, silicon and iron chlorophyll, protein, phosphates, formic acid and many other minerals. It is hardly surprising, then, that they should prove not only a good foliage feed for plants but an effective spray against mildew, black fly, aphides and plant lice. When you harvest nettles always cover yourself with protective clothing and wear heavy gloves. You can make a nutritious feed for your plants by soaking five or six handfuls of nettles in enough rainwater to cover them for two or three weeks. Strain and pour around the roots. I try to encourage my newly transplanted seedlings with a gentle dollop of this the moment they stand free in an open bed.

To make a foliage spray cover a generous handful of fresh nettles or 30 g (1 oz) of dried nettles with a litre (1¾ pints) of water and bring to the boil. Remove the pan from the heat immediately, cover tightly and cool. Strain and dilute with 3 litres ($5\frac{1}{4}$ pints) of water. Add a dessertspoonful of liquid soap (the kind you use to wash your dishes). This helps the spray stick to the foliage. Stir vigorously but not so much that you get a great froth of bubbles. Put into a spray gun or can. I found this particularly good for removing black fly from my stricken cherry tree one summer.

Yarrow Fertilizer

Yarrow is full of copper and contains traces of useful amounts of potash, phosphates, chlorides and lime. Lime is particularly important for herbs because it acts as a reagent and without it herbs cannot use the other nutritives in fertilizers. If your garden produces beautiful camellias, azaleas and rhododendrons, then you know it will need more lime added to the soil if you are to grow herbs successfully. Mix in the lime with equal quantities of magnesium carbonate and dig it into the soil. Then use a yarrow fertilizer to encourage your new seedlings. Simply follow the instructions for nettle fertilizer substituting yarrow. If it is to be used for root feeding rather than spraying omit the soap.

Garlic powder sprinkled among newly sown seeds keeps the birds from eating them as do powdered dried mugwort, rue and southernwood. If you sprinkle the seeds themselves with any of these dried herbs before planting and leave them for a few days to absorb their aromas it will prevent them being eaten underground by slugs. Of course, all these fertilizers and fungus and insect repellents can be used for herbs grown indoors. They should be put into a fine mist spray bottle and the foliage should be sprayed once a week until it drips to ensure good healthy growth.

Herb Gardens

Let your imagination inspire you as to what sort of herb garden you would like: formal or informal, artistic, segmented and neat or casual and carefree. You may even like to devote a corner to a wild herb garden if you have lots of space and let mullein, foxgloves, teasel, honesty and nettles run riot. Wood anemones, wild violets and woodruff could possibly be encouraged to grow in a moist, shady corner – the woodruff in my garden grows very satisfactorily beneath a large rosemary bush. The Elizabethans preferred the orderly surrounds of paradise gardens which they laid out in meticulous symmetrical patterns, symbolic of balance and harmony, in the centre of which stood the tree of life, cousin to the tree of knowledge from which Eve tempted Adam. It was symbolically represented by a fruit tree, shrub or a sundial. There were brick paths between the patterns of herbs, to enable the herbalist to walk right into the centre and have easy access to the herbs. You could make a simpler version of this by planning your herb garden in the shape of a Camembert cheese, each wedge separated by a path and containing a different herb. I must admit I have enjoyed a quiet laugh at some authorities, who advise utilizing an old cartwheel, for in this motorized age the odd discarded cartwheel is a rarity. You may be lucky enough to find them scattered all over the place but I have never encountered anything more exciting than old tyres and the inner tubes of bicycle wheels.

Herbs, given their few dislikes, will grow almost anywhere. A small bed only 4 m (4 yards) long by 1·5 m (1½ yards) wide will supply all your cosmetic as well as your culinary needs. Make sure when you plant them that tall herbs stand at the back and that shade-loving herbs enjoy some shelter near a wall or hedge. Medium-sized ones like mint, sage, thyme, salad burnet, tansy, bergamot and hyssop come next. Try to contain mint in a bowl or large terracotta pot just submerged beneath the surface, or wedge the mint round with roof slates, dug deep into the soil with the tops just apparent. Even using several large terracotta pots I still find my mints creeping over the edge and popping up in all sorts of unexpected places but this precaution does at least keep the problem in hand for a little while. Sow very short plants like chives and cowslips in the front.

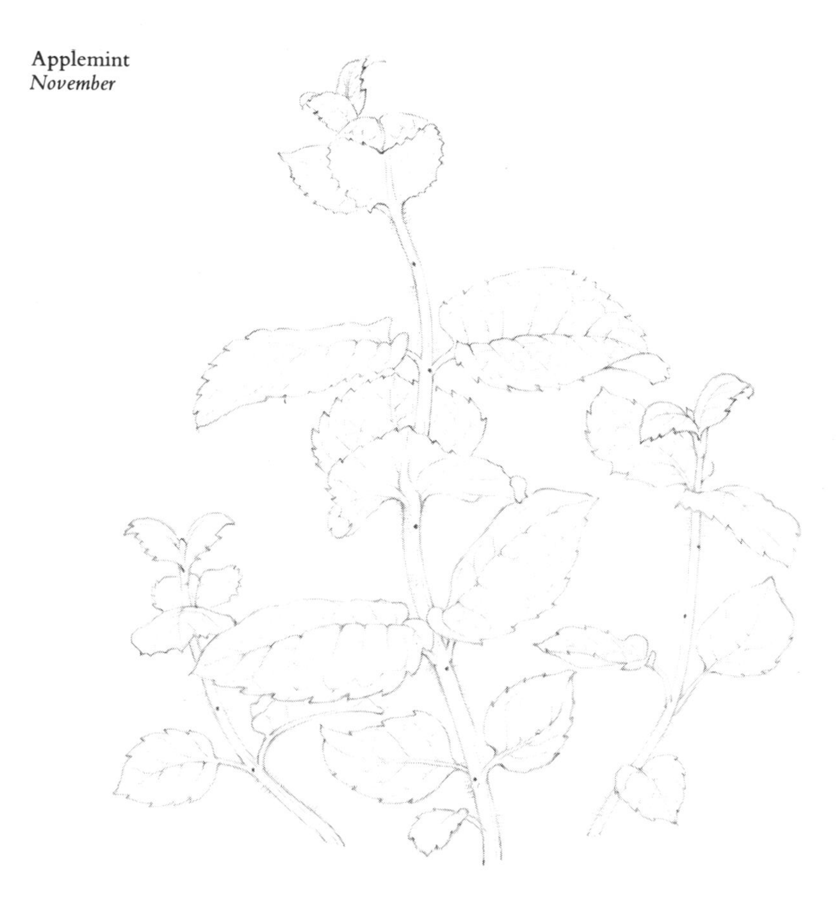
Applemint
November

Herb Lawns

In the Middle Ages imitations of natural meadows 'starred with a thousand flowers' were in vogue and very hard work they must have been too. They can still be seen depicted on medieval tapestries. These were succeeded by sweet-smelling chamomile lawns, and grass as we know it was considered a weed and therefore a pest. Nowadays, unless you want to spend hours fanatically weeding your lawn it is best to give in to a mixture of grass and weeds which, as I have already pointed out, are really only wild herbs. They are very useful cosmetically. White clover (*Trifolium repens*), suckling clover and yellow trefoil (*Trifolium dubium*), provide a permanent and perfectly balanced fertilizer for the lawn. Besides being a source of sodium clovers encourage and store the nitrogen-fixing bacteria in their root nodules, so that even in the driest summers there is a good supply of those elements necessary to keep the grass lush and brilliantly green. Yarrow, bursting with minerals, is another excellent lawn herb and chamomile provides calcium. Thyme's strong aromatic oil is a good bactericide. This herb lawn mixture was first evolved after the First World War by the Imperial War Graves Commission. It withstood the trampling of many thousands of visitors. Pennyroyal can also be added to this mixture but it will not stand too much trampling.

Indoors

Even if you live in a city it is still possible to grow some of your own herbs in tubs, window boxes and hanging baskets. Indoor herb growing is fairly simple. Do not squash your herbs into tiny pots; larger pots are preferable because they contain more soil, which keeps the moisture longer and contains more bacteria so the herbs come closer to their natural growing conditions. Choose a container with holes or slits underneath to allow any excess water to drain out. In Greece they utilize old oil drums and paint them white. They look most effective spilling over with red geraniums. Old cider barrels cut in half, if you can find them, or orange crates will do just as well as expensive terracotta pots, though I must admit the bright ochre of the pots is a lovely foil for the soft grey-green of the herbs inside them.

Use a well-balanced compost like John Innes No. 2 or one of the modern proprietary soil-less composts. Soil dug up from your garden will not do as it tends to encourage the growth of various fungi and sometimes becomes waterlogged. Water the herbs from below, using the saucer in which the pot stands, and throw out any surplus water after two hours. Do not fall into the trap of overwatering which tends to catch so many indoor gardeners, bent on killing with kindness. The top soil may very occasionally appear dry, in which case it should be watered sparingly from the top. Keep the room well-aired and do not put your herbs in draughts. Mint, woodruff, sweet cicely, lady's mantle, balm, lovage, houseleek and chervil grow quite well without direct sunlight, but other herbs need to be put on sunny window ledges and rotated from time to time to allow the whole plant to enjoy an equal share of the light. Pinch off the tops to encourage bushy growth and when you cut the herb for your use take only a few select sprigs here and there so that the plant does not get bald patches and look unbalanced.

Sweet Cicely
September

Herbs can be grown equally well in window boxes. Sir Hugh Platt, an Elizabethan who among his many other talents was a proficient gardener, advised: 'In every window you may make square frames either of lead or of boards well pitched within. Fill them with some rich earth and plant such flowers or herbs therein as you like best.' Lead won't do your plants any good and if the window box is wooden some sort of modern wood preservative might be more suitable than tar pitch. Place crocks over the drainage holes to prevent them blocking up. Fill with John Innes No. 3 compost and let it settle down for forty-eight hours. Herbs like balm, chives, cotton lavender, marjoram, nasturtiums, parsley, pennyroyal, sage, basil, thyme and winter savory are all suitable for window boxes and can last for some time without water. During the summer spray with your indoor sprayer in the cool of the evening and water from above as required.

Hanging baskets should be lined with a moisture-absorbing moss to prevent the soil inside falling through and they should contain a few lumps of charcoal which will help sweeten the mixture of peat and turf loam in the basket. Allow the soil to settle for a few days and plant the taller herbs in the centre and the smaller trailing ones on the outside. Do not expect to harvest many herbs from any of your indoor efforts. You will produce enough to make herbal tisanes, the odd flavoursome pinch for your cookery and enough for the occasional face mask, jar of cream and herbal toner. But you certainly will not be able to cull enough for something which requires a generous quantity of herbs like a herbal bath.

Propagation from Nursery Seedlings

If you are just beginning to grow herbs the best plan would be to find a good herb nursery and buy some potted seedlings from them. Some operate a mail order service. Once the herbs have four distinct leaves they can be moved to an open bed but make the transition gradual. Leave them outside in a sheltered spot for a week or two in order to get acclimatized. Then soak the seedling in its plastic pot in water (some come in plastic wrapping which can be subjected to the same treatment). Let the excess water drain out and carefully invert the pot, holding it with one hand and covering the top soil with the other, fingers slightly apart to allow the seedling to poke out between them. Squeeze the pot repeatedly until the herb and its rootlets embedded in the soil come out in one piece; alternatively, carefully peel away thc plastic wrapping. Then, keeping the herb firmly encased in its native soil, transplant it outdoors so that the bottom of the stem is a good 2½ cm (1 in.) below the surface. Water gently in the evening. If the seedling droops help it with a little natural fertilizer. Do not be afraid to talk to it and encourage it, it really does help. I was first instructed to talk to fruit bushes as I watered them when I spent a summer in California and as the result of my verbal encouragement (and doubtless the watering) they produced loads more fruit then usual. If you wriggle with embarrassment at the very concept then at least give your herbs the benefit of your loud, positive, encouraging thoughts. Plants, like people, like to be appreciated.

Propagation from Seed

This may sound obvious but always ensure your seed is fresh. Dusty, neglected packets unearthed from the back of some shelf are a waste of time and I have had a few disappointments buying seed of dubious character. You will notice by the instructions on the packet that most seed requires planting in March or April when the soil is just beginning to thaw. Help the soil along by pouring hot water over it before planting your seeds. This will speed up their germination. Do not, as I have seen some authorities advise – particularly to hurry along the eight-week germination period of parsley – use boiling water. This will only kill off the valuable living organisms in the soil. Parsley can be helped by soaking the seeds overnight in lukewarm water to soften the hard seed coats. Mix the seeds into a little sand before planting. This will help retain their precious moisture and deter greedy slugs. Sow in moist ground and water it gently afterwards with a rose attached to your can or hose. Take this precaution even after the seedlings have appeared, to save flattening them. Thin them out when they are 5 cm (2 in.) high.

Some of the less hardy herbs need to be started indoors. Wait until you can clearly see four young leaves, then proceed as with nursery seedlings. Some herbs can be propagated simply by splitting them. Chives, for example, can be divided and planted in smaller clumps in the autumn and in the spring and should be watered with yarrow fertilizer to prevent them turning yellow. Some can be taken indoors to ensure a constant supply, but again keep the soil well fertilized and only cut twice. Parsley will not stand cutting more than once in the winter.

Propagation by Cutting

Woody herbs like sage, lavender, rosemary and thyme respond well to this method. People with green fingers can achieve results simply by snapping off a twig and shoving it in the ground, but those of us who are all thumbs (like me!) need more accurate advice. Cut a 15-cm (6 in.) new sprout from a sturdy plant severing just below the leaf bud or stem joint so the twig has a heel. Place it in some water mixed with rooting compound and wait for the tiny rootlets to appear, then transplant outdoors being as gentle as you would with new seedlings. Strip off the lower leaves and water generously. Keep the foliage damp with a mist sprayer. You will find soft stemmed plants like mint and balm usually take a week or two to produce roots and woody ones like lavender may take nearly two months.

Alternatively, place the cuttings round the edge of a large terracotta pot filled with a mixture of one-third rooting compound, one-third sand and one-third peat moss. Once you can see strong leaf growth you will know they have rooted. Leave them for a week or two. Strip off the old leaves and transplant to an open bed.

Propagation by Layering

Many herbs which grow close to the ground can be propagated by layering. This is even simpler and surer than propagation by cutting. Just take one of the still-attached branches of the parent herb and bend it gently towards the earth. You may need to anchor it there with a U-shaped piece of wire. Then water generously to encourage root growth to spread down into the soil from the point where the plant touches it. After several weeks you will see a complete new plant forming and after six weeks you can sever it from its parent plant and transplant it. Balm, catmint, all scented geraniums, horehound, hyssop, marjoram, all the mints, rosemary, sage, winter savory and all the thymes respond well to this treatment.

Choosing your Herbs

The choice of herbs for your garden is entirely up to you, but it is advisable to read through the sections on skin care before going ahead to make sure you are cultivating the right herbs for your skin type. If you get swept away with enthusiasm, as I hope you will, and decide to treat your family and friends with your efforts then your selection of herbs will of course have to be much wider.

Symbiosis

Besides having a sympathetic attitude to your herbs you may notice many herbs enjoy a certain empathy and sympathy between each other. This is called 'plant symbiosis' and it is not at all fanciful. It is a proven fact and it would be as well to bear in mind the special relation some herbs have with each other and with vegetables and flowers. Chamomile is a superb plant nurse. Put near an ailing plant it will restore it to health and strength quite quickly, but it must not be left too long once the plant patient has recovered, otherwise this new lease of life is rapidly reversed. I have found that rue hates being near sage and basil, and if these herbs are all put in the same bed one or all of them tends to give up the ghost.

Borage gives strawberries an extra fillip. In fact borage with its generous supply of potassium, calcium and mineral salts which it releases into the soil is a helpful plant anywhere in your garden. Foxgloves stimulate the growth and endurance of neighbouring plants and a tea made from its leaves added to the water of flower arrangements will make them last longer. This seems much more acceptable than dosing the water with aspirin. African marigolds' fragrance is obnoxious to aphides and white fly and the excretion from their roots into the surrounding soil not only scares off root-lice but is absorbed by other plants so that they too are less attractive to pests. Garlic, chives and shallots are welcome neighbours to most plants except peas and beans which are noticeably retarded by their presence. Carrots become larger and tastier encouraged by friendly chives and shallots and leeks discourage carrot-fly pest. Roses grown near any member of the onion family suffer less from black spot and they have a particular affection for garlic. I have noticed it not only strengthens them but improves their scent. Parsley helps fend off aphis attacks on roses. In fact, the aromatic herbs tend to help all ailing plants and they have a repellent effect on many destructive insects above and below the ground, so be lavish with them. Hyssop is believed to encourage the growth of grape vines. Nettles grown with angelica, valerian, marjoram, sage and the mints noticeably increase the essential oil content of these plants and nettles and strawberries are good companions. Shakespeare noticed this centuries ago:

'The strawberry grows underneath the nettle,
And wholesome berries thrive and ripen best
Neighbour'd by fruit of baser quality.'
Henry V, Act I, Scene 1

Nettles, hyssop and rue all egg each other on to grow taller and greener. Fennel, on the other hand, retards the growth of beans. Symbiosis is even evident with stored fruits and vegetables: never store apples and potatoes together, for example. The apples will only taste flat and the potatoes will rot because apples exude ethylene gas which speeds up the growing process in potatoes.

I began my *Book of Herbal Beauty* with a quotation from William Turner which acknowledges far more eloquently than I am able to my debt to the authors of old herbals. The enthusiasm and delight expressed in them has proved infectious and I hope I have managed to instil a little of the same in you. However, library gardening is not enough. Therefore:

'I hope you will think it no dishonour to follow the steps of our grandsire Adam, who is commonly pictured with a Spade in his hand, to march through the Quarters of your Garden with the like Instrument, and there to rectify all the disorders thereof, to procure as much as in you lyes the recovery of the languishing Art of Simpling . . . There is no better way to understand the benefit of it, than by being acquainted with Herballs and Herbarists and by putting this Gentle and ingenious Exercise in practise.'

William Coles, *The Art of Simpling*, 1656

Botanical Index

As with any other science, nomenclature gets updated periodically. The names in this botanical index have therefore been checked against at least two sources.

Dock *Rumex alpinus*
Elder, European *Sambucus nigra*
Elecampane *Inula helenium*
Elm *Ulmus campestris*
Elm, Slippery *Ulmus fulva*
Eyebright *Euphrasia officinalis*
Fennel *Foeniculum vulgare*
Fern, Maidenhair *Asplenium trichomanes*
Fig *Ficus carica*
Gardenia *Gardenia* spp.
Garlic *Allium sativum*
Gentian, Spring *Gentiana verna*
Geranium, Common *geranium* spp.
Geranium, Scented *Pelargonium*
Ginseng, America *Panax quinquefolium*
Ground Elder *Aegopodium podagraria*
Hawkweed, Mouse-ear *Hieracium sylvaticum*
Hawkweed, Wood *Hieracium pilosella*
Hawthorn *Crataegus monogyna*
Heather *Calluna vulgaris*
Hemlock *Conium maculatum*
Hemp, Canadian *Apocynum cannabinum*
Hemp, Indian *Cannabis sativa*
Henbane *Hyoscyamus niger*
Henna *Lawsonia alba* or *Lawsonia inermis*
Hibiscus *H. rosa-sinensis*
Hollyhock *Althaea rosea*
Honeysuckle *Lonicera caprifolium*
Hop *Humulus lupulus*
Horseradish *Rorippa armoracia*
Horsetail *Equisetum arvense*
Hound's Tongue *Cynoglossum officinale*
Houseleek *Sempervivum tectorum*
Hyssop *Hyssopus officinalis*
Indigo *indigofera tinctoria*
Iris, Blue Flag *Iris versicolor*
Ivy *Hedera helix*
Ivy, Ground *Glechoma hederacea*
Jaborandi *Pilocarpus jaborandi*
Jasmine, Common White *Jasminum officinale*
Juniper *Juniperus communis*
Kelp, Irish Moss *Chonorus crispus*
Knot Grass *Polyganum aviculare*
Lady's Mantle *Alchemilla vulgaris*
Lady Smock (Cuckoo Flower *Cardamine pratensis*
Lavender *Lavendula officinalis*
Lettuce, Garden *Lactuca sativa*
Lettuce, Wild *Lactuca virosa*
Lily, Madonna *Lilium candidum*
Lime *Citrus aurantifolia*
Linden *Tilia europaea*
Linseed (Flax) *Linum usitatissimum*
Liquorice *Astragalus glycyphyllos*
Lovage *Ligusticum scoticum*
Lungwort *Sticta pulmonaria*
Lupin *Leguminosae*
Madder *Rubia tinctorum*
Mallow, Marsh *Althaea officinalis*
Marigold, Pot *Calendula officinalis*
Marjoram, Sweet *Origanum marjorana*
Marjoram, Wild *Origanum vulgare*
Meadowsweet *Filipendula ulmaria*
Melilot *Melilotus officinalis*
Mint, Pennyroyal *Mentha pulegium*
Mint, Peppermint *Mentha piperita*
Mint, Spear *Mentha viridis*
Mistletoe *Viscum album*
Motherwort *Leonurus cardiaca*
Mugwort *Artemisia vulgaris*
Mullein, Great *Verbascum thapsus*
Mustard, Black *Brassica nigra*
Mustard, White *Brassica alba* or *brassica hirta*
Myrrh *Commiphora myrrha*
Narcissus *Narcissus tazetta*
Nasturtium *Tropaeolum majus*
Nettle *Urtica dioica*
Nightshade, Deadly *Atropa belladonna*
Nutmeg *Myristica fragrans*

Olive *Olea europaea*
Orange, Bitter *Citrus vulgaris*
Orange, Sweet *Citrus aurantium*
Orchid *Orchidaceae*
Oregano *Origanum vulgare*
Orris root *Iris florentina*
Pansy *Viola tricolor*
Parsley *Petroselinum sativum*
Parsnip *Pastinaca sativa*
Pawpaw (Papaya) *Carica papaya*
Peach *Prunus persica*
Pimpernel, Scarlet *Anagallis arvensis*
Pine *Pinaceae*
Pineapple *Ananas comosus*
Pitcher Plant *Sarracenia purpurea*
Plantain, Common *Plantago major*
Poppy, Red *Papaver rhoeas*
Poppy, White *Papaver somniferum*
Potato *Solanum tuberosum*
Primrose *Primula vulgaris*
Privet, Common or Wild *Ligustrum vulgare*
Purslane *Portulaca sativa*
Quassia *Picraena excelsa*
Quince *Pyrus cydonia*
Radish *Raphanus sativus*
Rampion *Campanula rapunculus*
Raspberry *Rubus idaeus*
Rest Harrow *Ononis arvensis*
Rhubarb *Polygonaceae*
Rocket *Hesperis matronalis*
Rose *Rosaceae*
Rose, Apothecary *Rosa gallica*
Rose, Damask *Rosa damascena*
Rosemary *Rosmarinus officinalis*
Rue *Ruta graveolens*
St John's Wort *Hypericum perforatum*
Safflower *Carthamus tinctorius*
Saffron Crocus *Crocus sativus*
Sage *Salvia officinalis*
Sandalwood *Santalum album*
Savory, Summer *Satureja hortensis*
Savory, Winter *Satureja montana*
Scabious (Devil's Bit) *Scabiosa succisa*
Sea Holly *Eringium maritimum*
Sesame *Sesamum indicum*
Shepherd's Purse *Capsella bursa-pastoris*
Silverweed *Potentilla anserina*
Soapwort *Saponaria officinalis*
Solomon's Seal *Polygonatum multiflorum*
Sorrel, French *Rumex scutatus*
Sorrel, Wood *Oxalis acetosella*
Southernwood *Artemisia abrotanum*
Soy *Glycine soja*
Spurge, Spotted *Euphorbia maculata*
Storax (Styrax) *Liquidambar orientalis*
Strawberry *Frageria vesca*
Sunflower *Helianthus annuus*
Sweet Cicely *Myrrhis odorata*
Tansy *Tanacetum vulgare*
Teasel *Dipsacus sylvestris*
Thistle, Holy (Blessed) *Carbenia benedicta*
Thyme, Garden *Thymus vulgaris*
Thyme, Wild *Thymus serpyllum*
Turmeric *Curcuma longa*
Valerian *Valeriana officinalis*
Verbena, Lemon *Lippia citriodora*
Vervain *Verbena officinalis*
Vine *Vitis vinifera*
Violet, Dog *Viola canina*
Violet, Sweet *Viola odorata*
Walnut, Black *Juglans nigra*
Watercress *Nasturtium officinale*
Willow, White *Salix alba*
Wintergreen *Gaultheria procumbens*
Witchhazel *Hamamelis virginiana*
Woodruff *Asperula odorata*
Wormwood *Artemisia absinthium*
Yarrow *Achillea millefolium*

Appendix I

Ingredients which sometimes cause Allergic Reactions

agrimony
almond oil
arrowroot
birch bark and birch milk
buttercup
camphor
cocoa butter
corn starch
cowslips
daisy
essential oils of: basil
bay
bergamot
clary sage
neroli (orange blossom)
pennyroyal
peppermint
sage
spearmint
glycerine
golden seal
greater celandine
henna
honeysuckle
hops
horseradish
ivy
jaborandi
lanolin
laundry starch
lime blossom (if not used fresh)
linseed oil
lovage
mistletoe berries
mugwort
nasturtium
nettles
orris root
pansy
pawpaw
pennyroyal
pineapple
pine needles
plantain
primrose
quassia
quince seed
rue
Solomon's seal
southernwood
strawberries
sulphonated castor oil
tansy
tincture of benzoin
tincture of myrrh
white willow bark
wormwood
violet leaves
yellow sandalwood

Useful Names and Addresses

The Herb Society
34 Boscobel Place
London SW1 01–235 1530

Please enclose s.a.e. with all queries. The Society is by no means rich and would appreciate the gesture. They publish an excellent *Herbal Review* every quarter and have a wide network of regional organizers.

Herb Suppliers

Mr and Mrs Hugo
Ashfield Herb Nursery
Hinstock
Nr Market Drayton
Shropshire
Sambrook 392

Enclose s.a.e. for catalogue describing a wide range of herbs and seeds.

Dr Malcolm Stuart
Albion Botanicals Ltd
8 Grange Gardens
Cambridge
Cambridgeshire

Dr Stuart, formerly president of the Herb Society, supplies a wide variety of herb seeds which are of excellent quality.

Argyll Herbal Remedies
Coombe Wood
Winscombe
Somerset
Winscombe 3390

A good selection of herbal teas and herbal extracts.

Aromatic Oil Co
12 Littlegate Street
Oxford OX11 QT
Oxford 42144

A very large selection of superb essential oils available by mail order.

Baldwins
173 Walworth Road
London SE17
01–703 5550

Apart from a wide selection of dried herbs they carry a good stock of essential oils and pharmaceuticals.

Chase Compost Seeds Ltd
Benhall
Saxmundham
Suffolk
Saxmundham 2149

A limited supply of organically grown seeds.

Cowley Wood Conservation Centre
Parracombe
North Devon
Parracombe 200

Some herbs.

Culpeper, Ltd.
Hadstock Road
Linton
Cambridge
CB1 6NJ
Cambridge 891196

Culpeper also has branches in Brighton, Norwich and two branches in London. Enclose s.a.e. for mail order catalogue.

Daphne Ffiske Herb Nursery
2 Station New Road
Brundall
Norwich
Norfolk
Norwich 712137

Enclose 20 pence and s.a.e. for catalogue.

Gerard House
736b Christchurch Road
Boscombe
Bournemouth
Hants
Bournemouth 35352

Mail order service. Enclose s.a.e. for herb catalogue. Some essential oils stocked.

Hereford Herbs
Ocle Pychard
Herefordshire
Hereford 78379

An interesting supply of frozen herbs mainly supplied to the retail trade.

Hollington Nurseries Ltd
Woolton Hill
Newbury
Berks RG15 9XT
Newbury 253908

A good selection of herbs, plant pots and hanging baskets.

John Bell & Croyden
52–4 Wigmore Street
London W1H 0AU
01–935 5555

Mail order service. S.a.e. for catalogue unnecessary. Extremely good selection of essential oils, flower waters, tinctures, lanolin, cocoa butter, beeswax, castile soap in flakes and almost any other aids you may need including douches.

L'Herbier De Provence
341 Fulham Road
London SW10
01–352 0012

An excellent selection of really well dried herbs.

Lighthorne Herbs
Lighthorne Rough
Moreton Morrell
Warwickshire
Moreton Morrell 426

An excellent selection of herbs for wholesale.

Kitty Little Ltd
51 Shropshire Street
Market Drayton
Shropshire TF9 3DA
Market Drayton 3258

Enclose s.a.e. for free catalogue.

Manor House Herbs
Wadeford
Chard
Somerset
Chard 2213

Send s.a.e. for catalogue.

D Napier & Sons
17/18 Bristo Place
Edinburgh
Scotland
031–225 5542

Catalogue 25 pence.

Norfolk Lavender Ltd
Caley Mill
Heacham
King's Lynn
Norfolk PE31 7JE
Heacham 70384

Good quality lavender and essential oil of lavender.

Oak Cottage Herb Farm
Nesscliffe
Shropshire
Nesscliffe 262

Old Rectory Herb Garden
Ightham
Nr Sevenoaks
Kent
Borough Green 882608

An excellent selection of herbs. Catalogue 25 pence.

Madge Hooper
Stoke Lacy Herb Garden
Bromyard
Herefordshire
Burley Gate 232

A herb farm that has been established for many years.

Suffolk Herbs
Sawyers Farm
Little Conrad
Sudbury
Suffolk
Bures 227247

A good selection of organically grown herbs and seeds. Seeds only available by mail order, but open 9–5 every Saturday for visitors.

Valeswood Herb Farm
Little Ness
Shropshire
Baschurch 376

Enclose s.a.e. A good selection of herbs.

Woodlands Farm Nurseries
Broad Oak Road
Canterbury
Kent
0622 812491

For Advice on Organic Gardening

The Soil Association
Walnut Tree Manor
Haughley
Stowmarket
Suffolk IP14 3RS

Henry Doubleday Research Association
20 Convent Lane
Bocking
Braintree
Essex

Cosmetic Camouflage

The British Red Cross Society runs a highly specialized service using trained volunteer beauticians to teach hospital patients the art of cosmetic camouflage. They work under the umbrella of the Department of Health. For hospitals offering this service contact Red Cross Headquarters, 9 Grosvenor Crescent, London SW1.

There is also a Keromask Clinic in London which offers demonstrations on cosmetic camouflage and consultancies.
The clinic is at:
Innoxa (England) Ltd
Silver City House
62 Brompton Road
London SW1
01–581 3111

Suribachis

The following shops sell suribachis of various sizes:

London branches:
Notting Hill Gate – 4 Pembridge Road W11 01–221 5111
Kensington – 209 Kensington High Street W8 01–937 1440
South Kensington – 15 Old Brompton Road SW7 01–589 1725
Victoria – 157 Victoria Street SW1 01–828 0158
Croydon – 81 Whitgift Centre 01–680 1625

Other branches:
Birmingham – 47 North Court Birmingham
Shopping Centre 021–643 7961
Bournemouth – 79 Old Christchurch Road
Bournemouth 23691
Brighton – 18 Brighton Square The Lanes
Brighton 29658

Bibliography

I have found the first seven books particularly useful for identification. Don't restrict yourself to one. So much depends on individual taste and preference.

BENTHAM, G. and J. D. HOOKER, *Handbook of the British Flora*, 1887

BUTCHER, R. W. and L. HILL, *A New Illustrated British Flora*, vols. I and II, 1961

CLAPHAM, TUTIN and WARBURG, *Flora of the British Isles*, Cambridge University Press, 1959

GRIGSON, G., *The Englishman's Flora*, Paladin, 1958

HYDE, M., *Hedgerow Plants*, Shire Publications Ltd., Aylesbury, 1976

MARTIN, W. KEBLE, *The Concise British Flora in Colour*, Sphere Books, 1972

VEDEL, H. and J. LANGE, *Trees and Bushes in Wood and Hedgerow*, Methuen, 1960

ARBER, A., *Herbals: Their Origin and Evolution 1470–1670*, Cambridge, 1938

BACON, Sir FRANCIS, *Essays 'Of Gardens'*, 1625

BANCKES, RICHARD, *Herball*, 1515

BOYLE, Honourable R., *Medicinal Experiments*, 1718

CARTER, C., *The Compleat City and Country Cook*, 1732

CLARK, L., *Secrets of Health and Beauty*, Pyramid Books, New York, 1969

COCKAYNE, O., *Leechdoms, Wortcunning and Starcraft*, 1865

COGHAN, T., *The Haven of Health*, 1584

COLES, W., *The Art of Simpling*, 1656

CULPEPER, N., *Culpeper's Complete Herbal* (originally 1653), W. Foulsham & Co. Ltd.

DAVIS, A., *Let's Eat Right to Keep Fit*, Signet, New York, 1970

DIGBY, Sir K., *Receipts in Physick and Chirurgery*, 1668

DOGGETT, M., *Book of Receipts*, 1682

Egerton, MS. 2415

EVELYN, J., *Acetaria: A Discourse of Sallets*, 1699

FAIRFAX, M., *Still-Room Book*, 1630

GENDERS, R., *Herbs for Health and Beauty*, Robert Hale & Co., 1975

GERARD, J., *The Herball and Generall Historie of Plants*, 1597

Good Housewife's Handmaid, The. 1585

GRIEVE, Mrs M., *A Modern Herbal*, 2 volumes (edited by Mrs C. F.

Leyel), Hafner Publishing Co., New York, 1959
HARINGTON, Sir J., *The Englishman's Doctor. Or the Schoole of Salerne*, 1607
HIX, C., *Looking Good*, Hawthorne Books, New York, 1977
LANGHAM, W., *Garden of Health*, 1584
LAW, D., *A Guide to Alternative Medicine*, Turnstone Books, 1974
Leech Book of Bald. Anglo-Saxon. Believed to be A.D. 900–950
LEYEL, Mrs C. F., *The Truth About Herbs*, Culpeper Press, 1954
LOVELL, R., *A Compleat Herball*, 1659
LOWENFELD, C. and P. BACK, *The Complete Book of Herbs and Spices*, Pan, 1974
MARKHAM, G. *Countrey Contentments*, 1623
MESSEGUE, M., *Way to Natural Health and Beauty*, George Allen and Unwin Ltd., 1976
NOTT, J., *The Receipt Book*, 1723
PALAISEUL, J., *Grandmother's Secrets*, Penguin, 1976
PARKINSON, J., *Paradisi in Sole Paradisus Terrestris*, 1629
PHARMACY MEDICAL RECEIPTS. Sloane MS. 782, XVII century
PHILBRICK, H. and R. B. GREGG, *Companion Plants*, Stuart and Watkins, 1967
PLATT, Sir H., *Delightes for Ladies*, 1594
PUGHE, J., *The Physicians of Mydelvai*, 1861
RAM, W., *Ram's Little Dodeon*, 1606
RIMMEL, E., *Book of Perfumes*, 1865
ROHDE, E. S., *Herbs and Herb Gardening*, Medici Society, 1936
A Garden of Herbs, Dover Publications, New York, 1969
ROSE, G., *A Perfect School of Instructions for Officers of the Month*, 1682
ROSE, J., *Herbs and Things*, Grosset and Dunlap, New York, 1977
RUTLEDGE, D., *Natural Beauty Secrets*, Avon Books, New York, 1966
SHIRLEY, J., *The Accomplished Ladies Rich Closet of Rarities*, 1715
Sloane MS. 1829, XVII century
Sloane MS. 2552
TISSERARD, R. B., *The Art of Aromatherapy*, C. W. Daniel Co. Ltd., 1977
Toilet of Flora, 1779

Index